# AIDS Updates - Recent Advances and New Perspectives

*Edited by Samuel Ikwaras Okware*

Published in London, United Kingdom

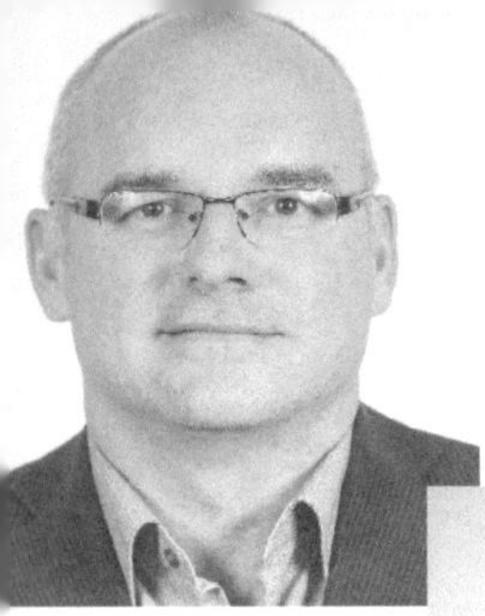
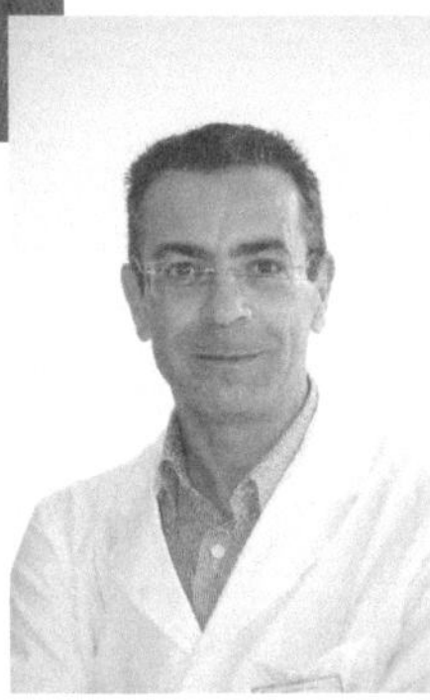
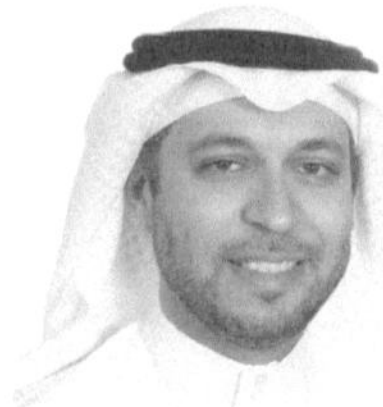
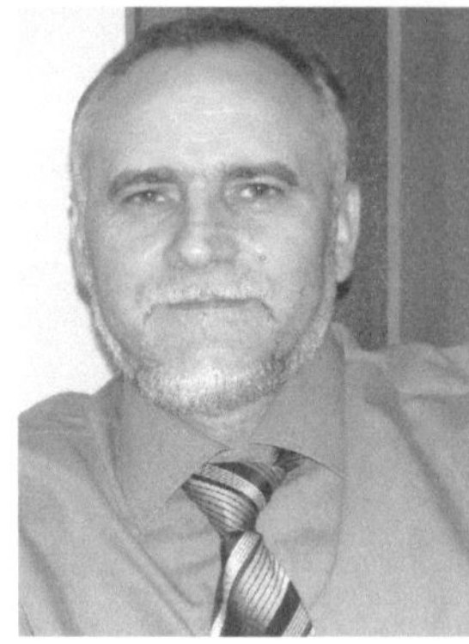
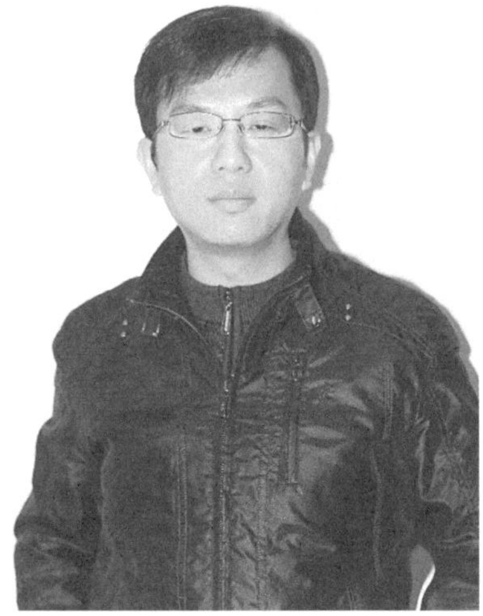
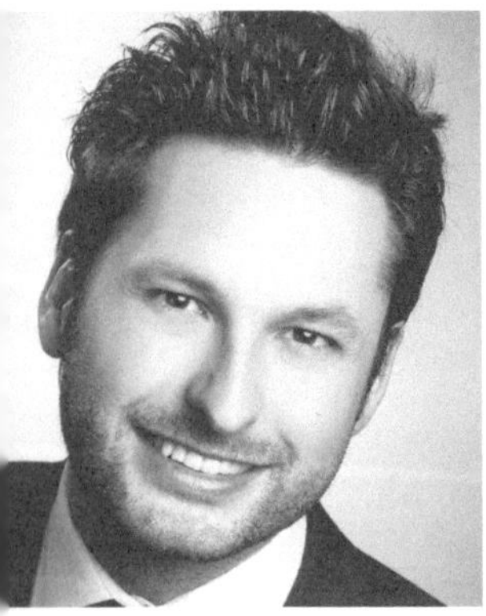
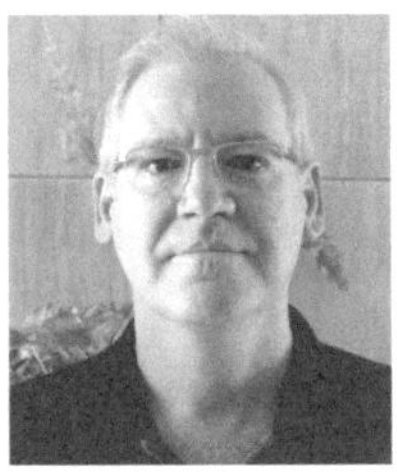

IntechOpen

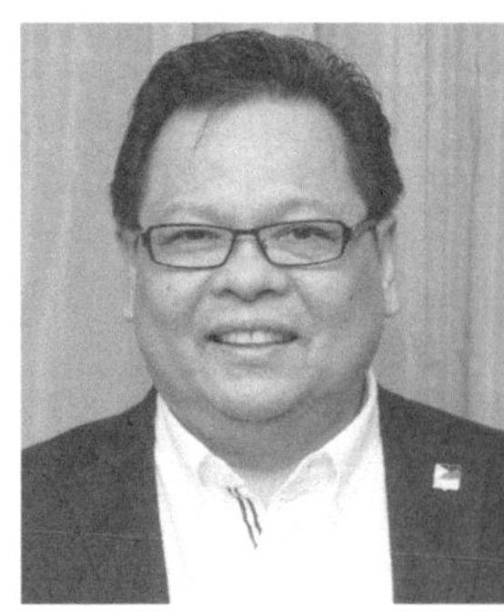
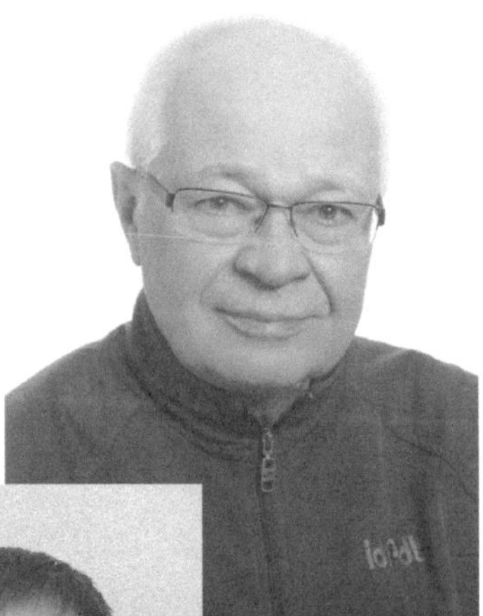
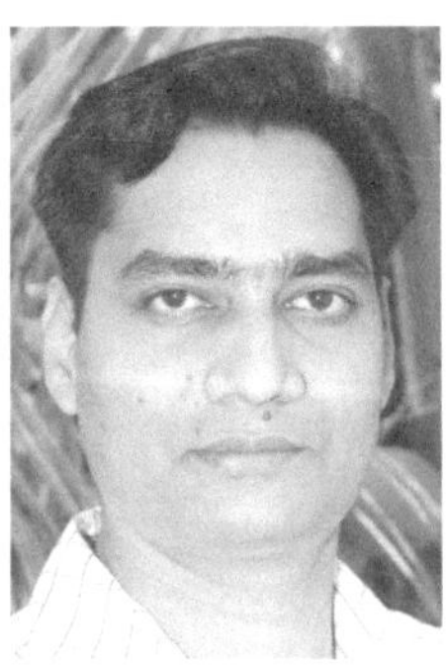
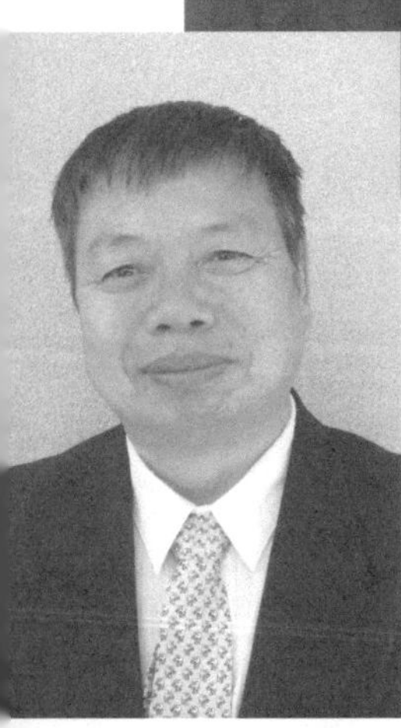
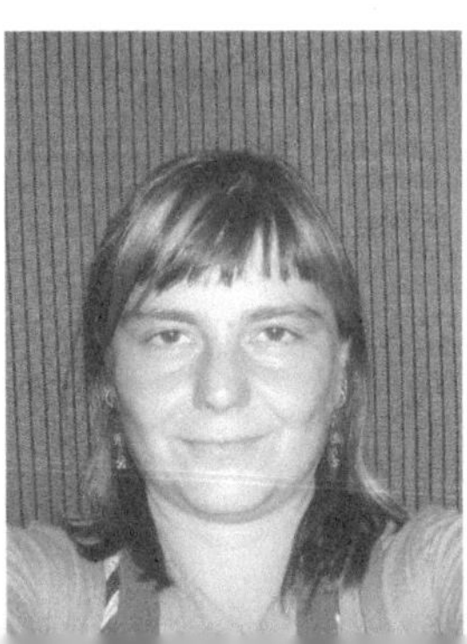
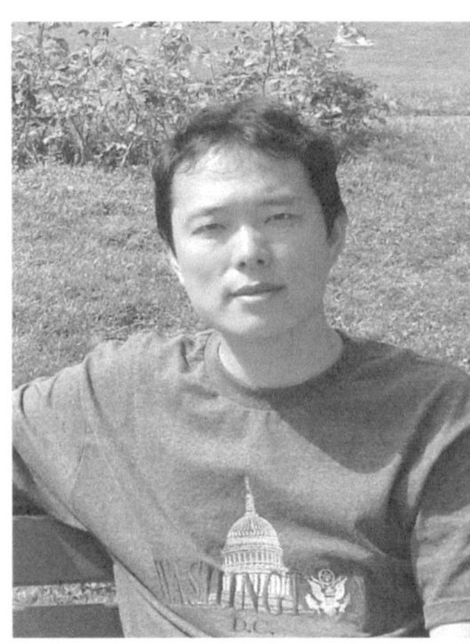

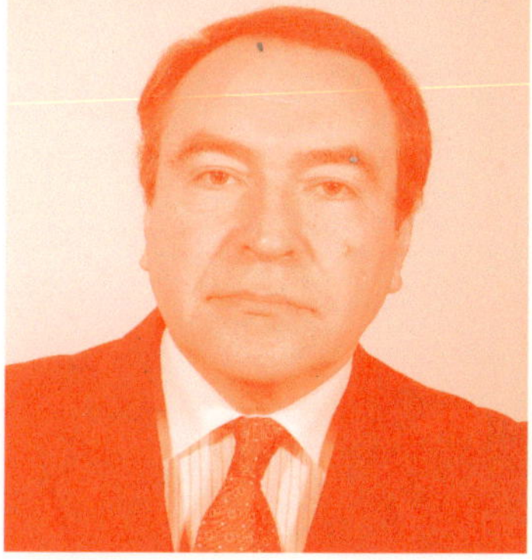

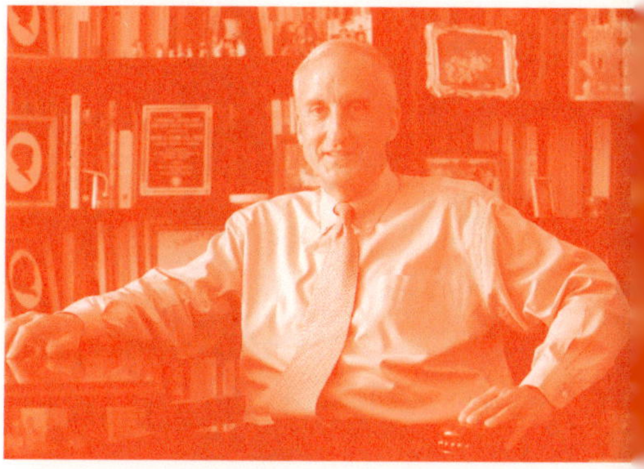

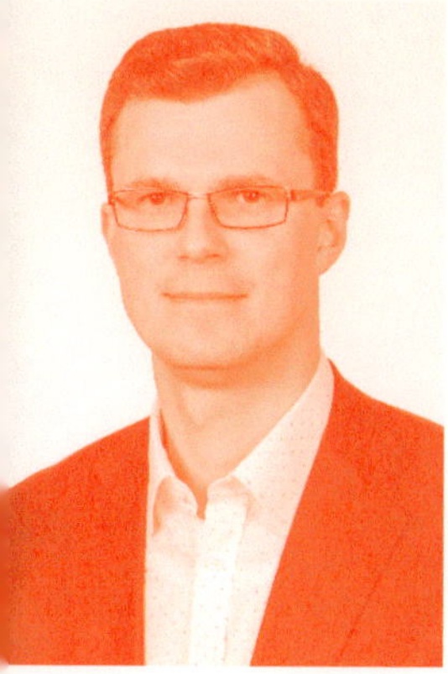

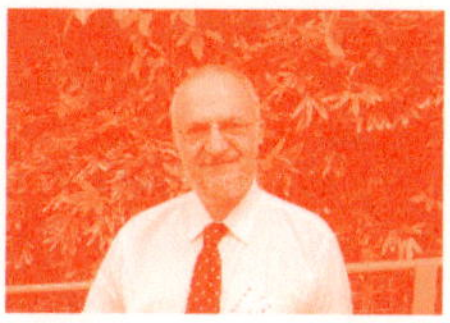

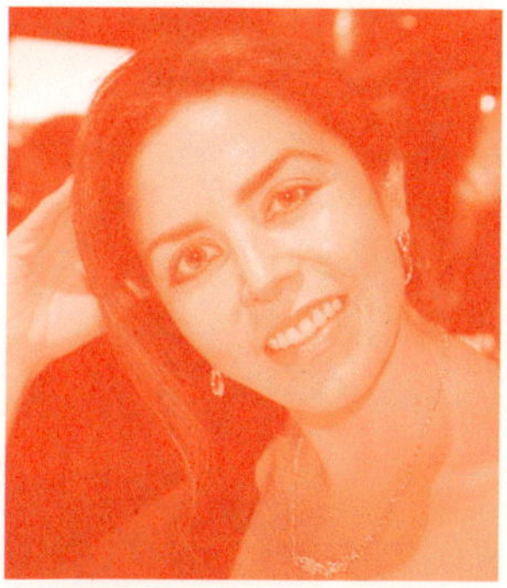

*Supporting open minds since 2005*

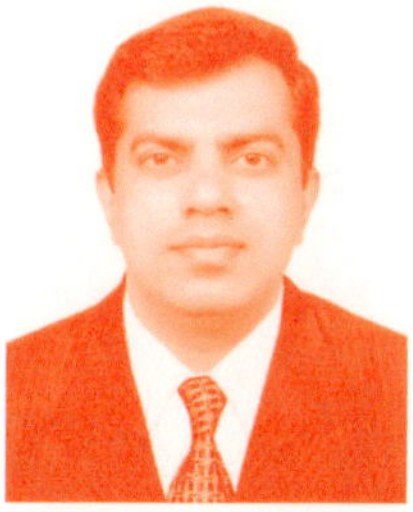

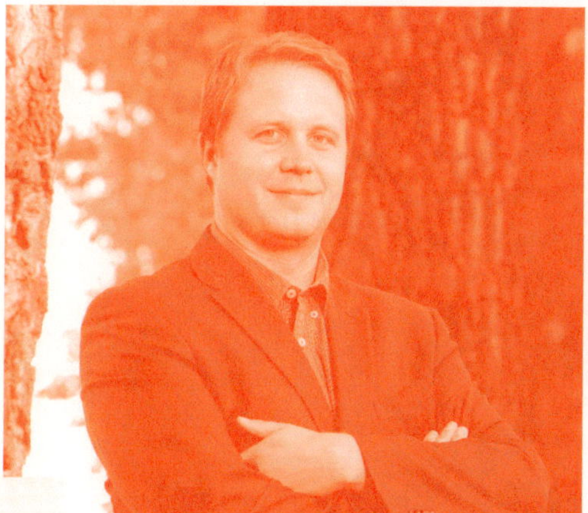

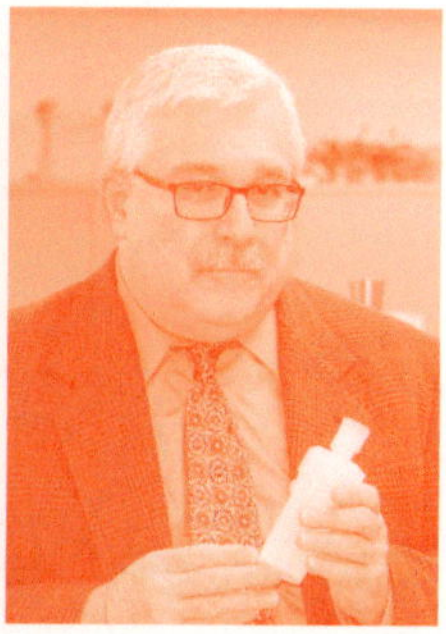

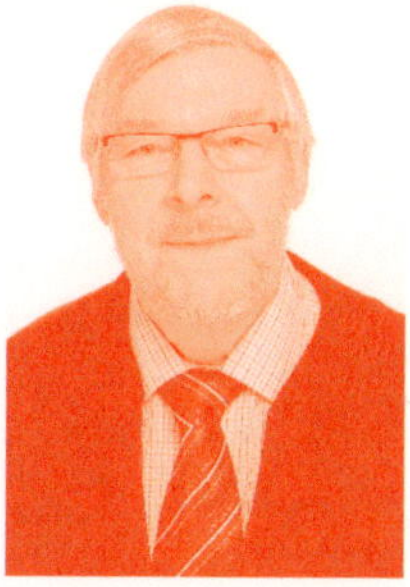

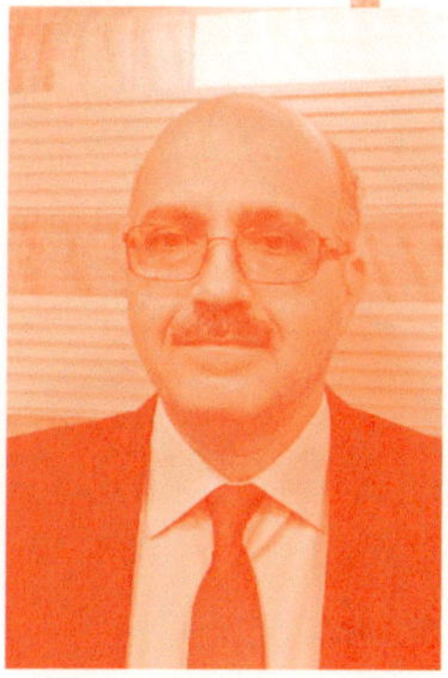

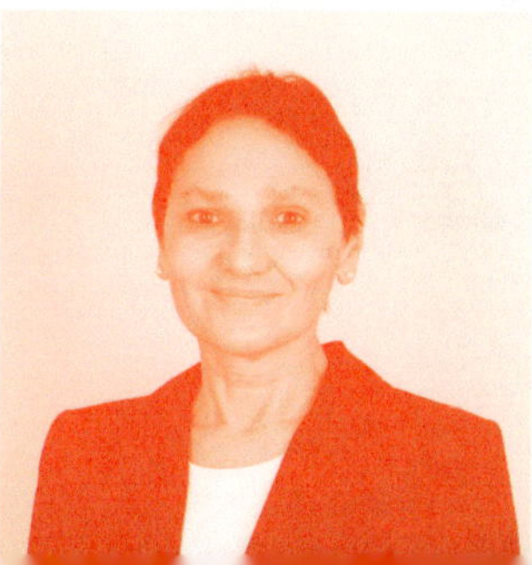

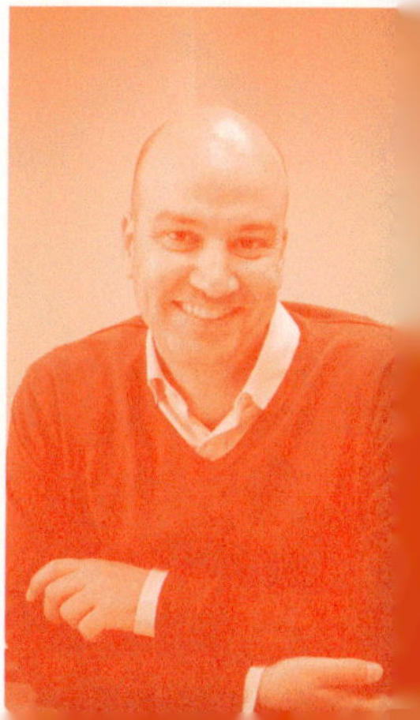

AIDS Updates - Recent Advances and New Perspectives
http://dx.doi.org/10.5772/intechopen.91514
Edited by Samuel Ikwaras Okware

Contributors
Fausta Mosha, Marcela Gómez-Suárez, Liza Conyers, Jen Yung-Chen Chiu, Sergio Rueda, Mark Misrok, Erin McKinney-Prupis, Vickie Lynn, Inampudi Sailaja, Manoj Kumar Baghel, Ivvala Anand Shaker, Adamu Muhammad Muhammad Hamid, Godwin Matthew Matthew Sule, Samuel Ikwaras Okware



First published in London, United Kingdom, 2021 by IntechOpen
IntechOpen is the global imprint of INTECHOPEN LIMITED, registered in England and Wales, registration number: 11086078, 5 Princes Gate Court, London, SW7 2QJ, United Kingdom
Printed in Croatia

British Library Cataloguing-in-Publication Data
A catalogue record for this book is available from the British Library

Additional hard and PDF copies can be obtained from orders@intechopen.com

AIDS Updates - Recent Advances and New Perspectives
Edited by Samuel Ikwaras Okware
p. cm.
Print ISBN 978-1-83969-358-8
Online ISBN 978-1-83969-359-5
eBook (PDF) ISBN 978-1-83969-360-1

# Meet the editor

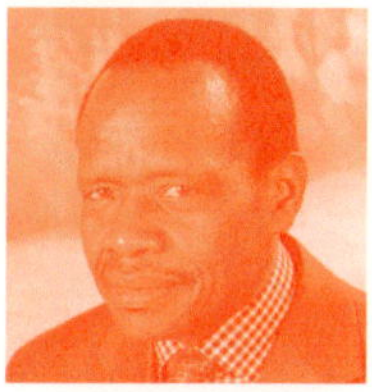

Samuel Okware is a public health specialist, epidemiologist, and lecturer. He obtained his Ph.D. in Emerging Infections from the University of Bergen, Norway. He pioneered the earliest HIV/AIDS investigations and work that contributed to major declines in HIV prevalence in the country. He led the national response that contained a large Ebola outbreak. He heads the Uganda National Health Research Organization, which regulates health research, and has held senior positions in the Ministry of Health, including Emergency Preparedness and Response. He was a consultant and a member of the WHO Expert Committee on Research and Development. He published several papers on communicable diseases and edited several books on HIV/AIDS and Ebola. He received several awards for his contribution to public health.

# Contents

# Preface

This book reviews some aspects of the global response to HIV/AIDS by select countries that have made significant progress in HIV prevention and control. It also examines emerging challenges and opportunities in the implementation of some of the initiatives discussed.

The first section discusses challenges and opportunities in the implementation of global strategies. Chapter 1 presents an overview of the earliest AIDS control program associated with success. It demonstrates details and examines the program's positive elements in reducing HIV prevalence and incidence. It also demonstrates the vital role of community mobilization countrywide in generating positive trends and HIV reductions at the national level. Chapter 2 reviews the critical role of the media as a major source of information for national programs. It examines challenges in the media within the context of societal perceptions and new communication technologies. It also takes a look at media exposure and its participation in HIV/AIDS prevention. Chapter 3 elaborates the key role of sexual and reproductive health as an entry point for prevention and control of HIV/AIDs especially in women living with HIV/AIDS. Sexual and reproductive health is critical in the implementation of national strategies, and this chapter discusses challenges for young women. A review of the central role of sexual and reproductive health in consolidating human rights-based program proposes additional suggestions to address gender balance and participation. Alternative guidelines based on new evidence for a woman-centered approach are suggested. The new approach assures reliable access to health and family-friendly services. Barriers to antiretroviral treatment at the community level are discussed and suggestions are made for improvement. New guidelines are proposed to provide a tool to help countries plan, develop, and monitor progress to promote gender equity and human rights.

The second section reviews treatment and improved opportunities. Chapter 4 discusses the determinants of adherence to antiretroviral therapeutic regimes among people with HIV/AIDS in select health facilities. It demonstrates the value of monitoring and determining the viral load to support adherence verification. It also discusses how to overcome barriers. Chapter 5 on nanotechnology demonstrates how new technologies can improve the effectiveness of antiretroviral treatment. It examines how opportunities offered by nanotechnology-based drug delivery systems can improve antiviral drug compliance and effectiveness. Some discussions are made on how nanotechnology offers better manufacturing and delivery processes. The chapter explains how nanomaterial drugs react directly to the targeted cells or tissues and offer a better and more effective healing effect. It describes in detail the different nanosystems that can be utilized. Chapter 6 discusses employment as a social determinant of HIV care and preventive outcomes. It also discusses HIV/AIDS as a chronic disease. As such, people living with HIV/AIDS must return to work and be integrated into the workforce. The chapter recommends integrating employment services within future HIV/AIDS programs. It also suggests and recommends client-focused work models for integrating employment as a social determinant in HIV/AIDS programs.

As we look towards our goal of HIV elimination by 2030, let no one be left behind as we take advantage of emerging opportunities, notwithstanding the impact of COVID 19, which has undermined the achievements in HIV/AIDS control, as outlined in the first chapter.

This book contains valuable knowledge and experiences from experts worldwide.

I thank the authors for their contributions. I also thank Author Service Manager Dolores Kuzelj at IntechOpen for her invaluable support and assistance.

**Dr. Samuel Ikwaras Okware Ph.D.**
Director General,
Uganda National Health Research Organisation,
Entebbe, Uganda

Section 1

# Updates in HIV/AIDS - Challenges and New Opportunities

Chapter 1

# Review of Social Challenges of Heterosexual Transmission of HIV/AIDS in Uganda

*Samuel Ikwaras Okware*


## Abstract

This Chapter reviews and discusses the experiences of Uganda and the lessons learnt during the successful implementation of its HIV/AIDS Control Program. The major mode of transmission was by the heterosexual route. Control measures thus emphasized behavior change and sexual discipline that promoted faithfulness and monogamous sexual relationships. This chapter examines the factors responsible for the positive outcomes in the implementation of the national AIDS control strategy. The review is based on literature, reports and personal experience. The Uganda Program AIDS in the Ministry of Health (MOH) was one of the earliest AIDS Control Programs in the world. A cumulative total of nearly 2 million people have been infected since the onset of the outbreak in 1982. Some one million HIV related deaths also occurred. When the National AIDS Control Program was initially rolled out in the country there was no cure and the disease was like a death sentence. The available evidence then demonstrated heterosexual transmission as the major mode of spread. Interventions based on the promotion of Abstinence, Being faithful, and Condom use (ABC strategy) were the main components of the strategy in the public campaigns. This complex disease also impacted society and the social fabric deeply. The activities were expanded to include the socio and economic dimensions of HIV/AIDS. Later on the combination strategy integrating biomedical and social behavior change strategies offered new and more encompassing opportunities. The introduction of the antiretroviral therapy (ART) and availability of simplified tests for detection of the viral load status improved treatment and restored hope. Social support and programs for reduction of stigma opened up participation by people living with HIV/AIDS. A community based intersectoral and decentralized strategy reached every village and assured community engagement and involvement. Drastic and steady declines in prevalence and incidence followed. Cases have been declining steadily and prevalence and incidence rates continue to drop and reverse the HIV status in the country. Community Engagement strategy to promote monogamous sexual behavior and the introduction of the highly active retroviral treatment significantly consolidated to the successful outcomes.


**Keywords:** HIV, Uganda, Prevention, social, challenges, community, success

## 1. Introduction

The Uganda model of HIV/AIDS prevention was often mentioned as a success story [1–6]. It was the first AIDS Control program in Africa. The Human Immunodeficiency

Virus (HIV) is a virus that attacks the body's immune system. It leads to Acquired Immunodeficiency Syndrome (AIDS), an unprecedented pandemic. HIV is a slow infection that may cause AIDS. However, the majority of People Living with HIV/AIDS (PLWHA) are asymptomatic. Heterosexual transmission is responsible for nearly 90% of the transmission [7–9] in Uganda.

The aim of This Chapter is to review and discuss the factors that influenced the success of the Ugandan AIDS/HIV Control Program. It examines the historical perspectives and outcomes by desk and literature reviews. Following the implementation of the ABC strategy, sharp declines in HIV prevalence were reported. From 1990 to 2000 HIV prevalence dropped from 18% in the 1990s to 6% over a ten-year period [1, 10]. In 1982 the first cases of HIV HIV/AIDS were reported in Rakai district of Uganda on the border with Tanzania. It was then referred to a "Slim Disease" because of the extreme wasting resulting from persistent fever and diarrhea. The local villagers believed it to be due to witchcraft as it affected mostly the rich and their spouses. Orphans were left helpless and many carried the family burden. The epidemic emerged at a time when the health system and services had been severely disrupted by years of insurgency. Cases were doubling every six months. The infection spread quickly along trade routes. When truck drivers and sex workers got infected they easily spread infection in urban areas. The rural communities initially were less affected. In urban areas the prevalence among antenatal mothers was 30% and the rural communities were less affected at just 3% in 1990. The mother to child transmission was less than 10%. Heterosexual transmission therefore remained the major route of infection [8, 11, 12].

The national response was organized and led by HE the President of Uganda. An intersectoral Committee of the Cabinet developed and executed one national joint plan across the sectors, ministries, departments and agencies. Each sector then developed their HIV strategies and work plans which were implemented in a decentralized approach. In 1992 coordination was shifted from the Ministry of Health (MoH) to the Uganda AIDS Commission (UAC) secretariat in the office of the President. Similar coordinating frameworks were then repeated at district, county sub county, parish and community levels. All these structures supported the National Strategic Plans (NSP) which was a decentralized and multisectoral response with emphasis on community participation. Maximum community involvement was the pillar to the approach for the prevention of the heterosexual transmission [5, 8, 9, 13] The program was supported by several bilateral and international partners, principally the United States of America, United Kingdom and several countries in the European Union in an arrangement led by the World Health Organization (WHO) and later by the Joint United Nations Program on HIV/AIDS (UNAIDS) [14]. UNAIDS leads and inspires the world to achieve its shared vision of zero new infections by 2030. Many lessons were learnt which have formed a basis for other emerging and remerging outbreaks.

## 2. The ABC strategy

Heterosexual transmission was the major mode of transmission and this was the focus of the national response. The ABC strategy in Uganda is cited positively for HIV prevention and control. The promotion of Abstinence, Being Faithful and Condom use (ABC Strategy) were critical components to HIV/AIDS prevention and control. The ABC Strategy were the key interventions to promote morality and reducing cases in the early years [2, 5, 11]. Primary abstinence, "A" occurs when a young person has never had sex. Secondary abstinence is when an adult delays sexual activity after initiation. Studies by the Medical Research Council

AIDS studies in Uganda demonstrated the protective value of primary abstinence. However this protection could last up to the age of 19 years, depending on one's current sexual behavior. Between 20 and 24 years there was no correlation between those who had delayed age of sexual debut and those who did not [15]. Abstinence has been improving as the age of sex debut dropped to 14 years from 17 years [16]. Being Faithful is practicing sex with one partner in a lifelong relationship. However, polygamy still exists in many communities in Uganda. In some polygamous marital relationships there are no clear boundaries of monogamy. The contribution of faithfulness is indirectly related to total fertility patterns. Total fertility rate in Uganda is six meaning that a mother may produce that number of children on average. The fertility has remained stagnant. This presumably may imply that women today are indulging in the same numbers of unprotected sexual contacts but with fewer partners than before, thereby yielding fewer new infections. It is plausible that although these women are having the same number of sexual contacts, they are doing so with fewer men.

## 3. Condoms

Correct and consistent use of male condom offers some degree of protection from HIV and other sexually transmitted infections [17, 18]. Uptake in the Uganda male has remained low but varied over the years [9, 16, 19]. In urban areas the demand for condoms is high. Local norms, high costs and stigma also impact access to condoms. Religious organizations claim that condom messages offer conflicting messages that undermine the moral standards of monogamous relationships. Others perceive that it promotes promiscuity. Condom uptake has since been scaled up and is a regular component of the National AIDS Control Program. Condom use has increased from 5% in the 1990s to 32% in 2019 [19, 20] The contribution of condoms in the reduction of the observed HIV infections is not clear. Most of the declines in HIV infections occurred long before the year 2000 when condom availability and use was still very limited [6]. That view then suggests that probably Abstinence and "Being Faithful" contributed the most in the early HIV declines. There are groups for which condoms remain a necessity. Discordant PLWHA will need condoms. Condoms are required during voluntary testing and counseling. Discordant married couples need condoms even in monogamous relationships. Promiscuity can be a problem even in marriage. A recent survey revealed that about 4% of married respondents admitted having a regular partner outside marriage for more than 12 months [16, 19]. Commercial sex workers, both formal and informal are very mobile. And have high HIV prevalence rates, often as high as 60%. Their work carries a very high risk of HIV acquisition. Sexually transmitted diseases are prevalent in these communities. Surveys show that 17% of women and 5% of men were infected [16, 19].

## 4. Trends in HIV prevalence

Uganda's population in 2021 is estimated at 41 million with a growth rate Of 3.02%. In 1986, the population was 15 m with the same growth rate [21–23]. About 80% live in rural areas while 20% reside in urban areas. The country has a predominantly young population: nearly 50% are below the age of 19 years [5, 21, 24]. The recent surveys indicate that about 1.4 million people in Uganda are living with HIV/AIDS [5, 19, 21] . HIV prevalence been declining steadily from 6.6% in 2010 to 6.1% in 2015 and 5.8% in 2020 (**Figure 1**) [25]. Similar trends over the last two

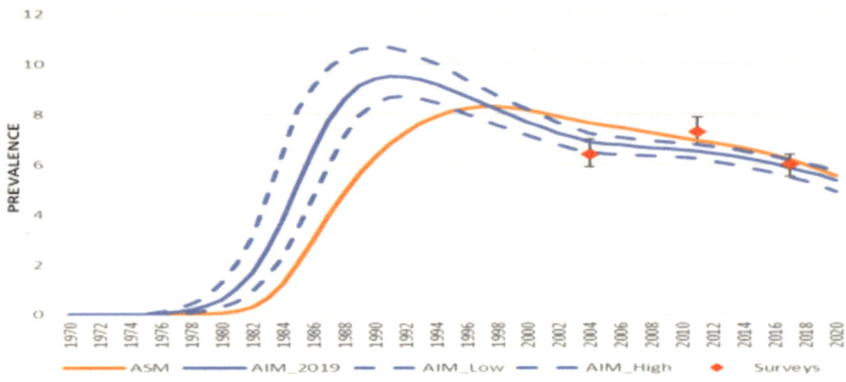


**Figure 1.**
*Trends in HIV prevalence among 15–49 year olds between 1970 and 2020. Source: Epi-data 1990–2020. In: AIDSinfo [database]. 17 may 2019–2021 Jan 2020. Geneva: UNAIDS; updated 30 June 2020 (http://aidsinfo.unaids.org/) [25].*

decades has been observed in the population [1, 12, 16, 26]. Even among the high risk groups, the burden is reducing. For instance, rates among commercial sex workers' declined from 68 to 37% between 1988 and 2020 [19, 27]. The age of sexual debut too reduced from 18 to 15 years. The number of sexual partners has also declined by half. Knowledge about HIV/AIDS remains high at 87% according to surveys [10, 12, 19]. The rural areas show the lower rates of about 2.0% during the period. Urban areas on the other hand have much higher prevalence rate of 7.5%. New infections too have declined by 62% from 3.19 in 2010 to 1.93 in 2015 and 1.3 in 2020 per 1000 persons (**Figures 2** and **3**) [25]. In 2019 some 53,000 new infections were recorded, compared with 67,000 in 2015, of which 5,700 children and 28,000 were among women. Females are infected four fold than males. Among antenatal mothers prevalence declined from 33% to less than 10% between 1990 and 1995. Among the general population there were significant similar declines - from 18 to 6% Mother to child transmission too has greatly declined by nearly 90% [6, 9]. Mortality rates too due to HIV/AIDS declined from about 53,000 in 2010 to 21,000 in 2019. AIDS-related deaths too declined over the past decade to approximately 21,000 in 2019 (compared to 29,000 in 2015 and 53,000 in 2010 (**Figure 4**) [12, 20, 25]. Males are more affected and their treatment adherence is lower. Some 70% of people living with HIV/AIDS were on antiretroviral treatment in 2020. Stigma generally has declined from 4.5% in 2013 to 1.3 in 2019 according to a National Study on Stigma Index [28, 29]. However,

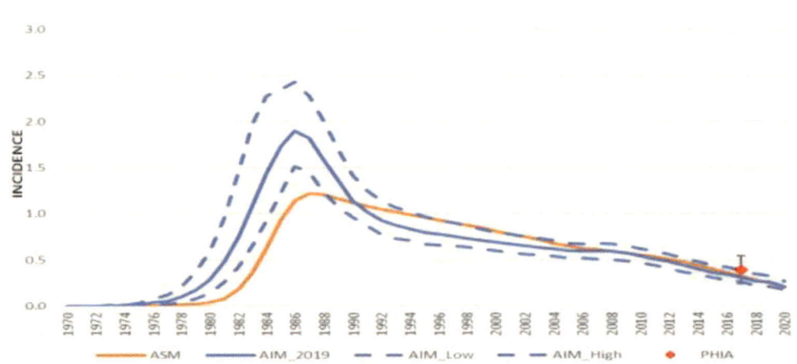


**Figure 2.**
*Trends in HIV incidence among 15–49 year olds between 1970 to 2020. Source: Epi-data 1990–2020. In: AIDSinfo [database]. 17 may 2019–2021 Jan 2020. Geneva: UNAIDS; updated 30 June 2020 (http://aidsinfo.unaids.org/) [25].*

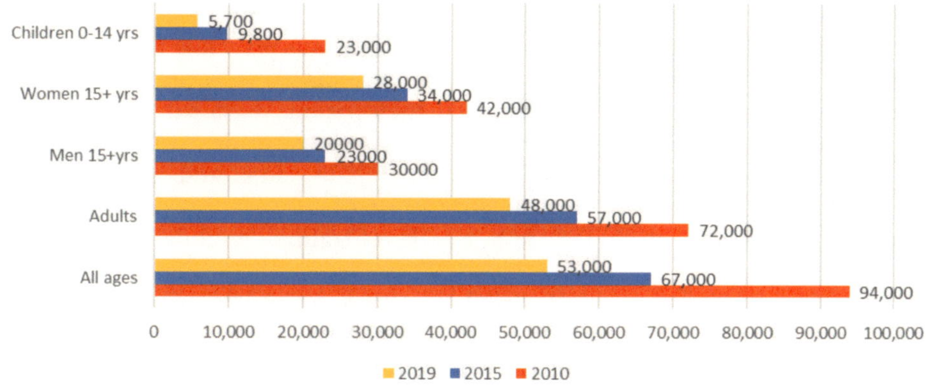


**Figure 3.**
*Trends in estimated new HIV infections by age and sex. Source: Epi-data 1990–2020. In: AIDSinfo [database]. 17 may 2019–2021 Jan 2020. Geneva: UNAIDS; updated 30 June 2020 (http://aidsinfo.unaids.org/) [25].*

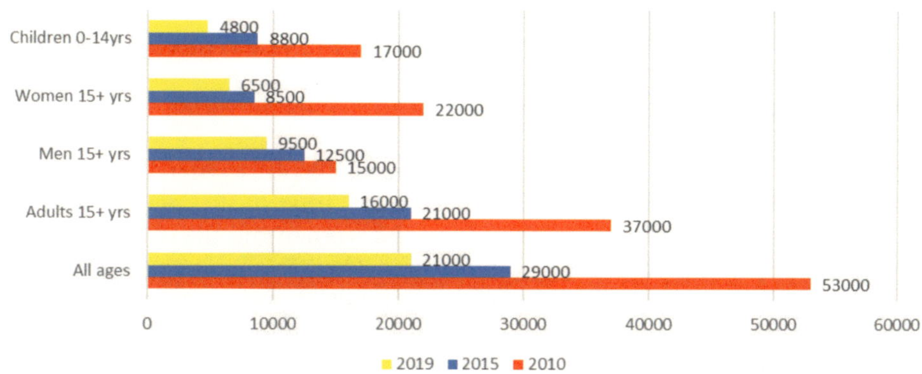


**Figure 4.**
*Trends in estimated numbers of AIDS-related deaths. Source: Epi-data 1990–2020. In: AIDSinfo [database]. 17 may 2019–2021 Jan 2020. Geneva: UNAIDS; updated 30 June 2020 (http://aidsinfo.unaids.org/) [25].*

some obsolete legislation in the Penal Code which criminalizes sex workers and same sex sexuality is yet to be repealed. Legal and policy changes should be made to reduce stigma and address human rights concerns.

Despite progress, some social and economic barriers persist. Structural elements such as gender inequality, economic inequities, cultural barriers and thinly veiled prejudices continue to undermine the target goals. It is not therefore surprising that new infections are highest among Adolescent Girls and Young Women (AGYW). Gender based violence is high especially during the COVID 19 lockdown restrictions. Poverty leads to social exclusion of women and limits access to social services. The rise of alcohol consumption and drug use has also been reported in these age group [28, 29].

## 5. Public education

Creating awareness about HIV/AIDS was the key for community participation and public education. Fear was used first as a deterrent but the people became insensitive to frightful images. Later the program embarked on a softer approach which targeted specific groups, with specific packages for the public, religious and nongovernmental organizations, schools and political cadres. The media campaign used elders, musicians, opinion leaders for mobilization. Intervention packages for the illiterate communities were also developed. The public and community based networks were happy with "Love Carefully". The religious preached the "Love Faithfully" message. The schools taught "Abstinence" as their major intervention. The children in turn conveyed the message to their parents. Basic infection control supplies and palliative drugs were included in the packages as part of home based care. Additional mobilization through entertainers, musicians, and other individuals with influence was carried out. The chairperson of the village coordinated this decentralized approach, strengthened by a series of training modules including the training of trainers.

The ABC strategy addressed the drivers of this route and contributed to the success and reduction of HIV infection in the initial phase. Later the three components were strengthened by the combination strategy which blended the biological components with behavior change package. The full introduction of antiretroviral therapy leveraged prevention and undetectable viral loads greatly reduced the risk of transmission [14]. The 90–90-90 Strategy involving test and treat was optimized combination strategies. HIV related mortality reduced by between 40 and 60% [16].

## 6. Needs of the young population

Uganda has a young population in which almost 50% are aged 0-19 years. This is the domain of turbulent sexual experiences. Other social determinants had to be tackled especially among the adolescent women and the youth. A study revealed key populations fuelling new infections. Therefore, among key vulnerable groups identified were adolescent girls and young women. Often some are coerced to exchange sex for money or other incentives. While the national HIV prevalence rates in the general population has declined, the prevalence rates in young women has remained higher at 7.4% compared to men at 4.3% [16, 20, 25]. These are very mobile groups. In a recent study assessing the movements of young commercial sex worker in Central Uganda, it was reported that over 81% reported different operating work sites many miles apart for their trade, thus increasing the geographical risk of transmission. While PrEP should be included in combination package for adolescents and young people, the programs should at the same time address the potential risks against other sexually transmitted infections and unwanted pregnancies [30].

Community engagement strategies must be strengthened to enable communities get involved in the provision of sustained services.

## 7. Needs of the elderly clients

The 90–90-90 strategy applies well for the relatively young groups, but does not fully meet the needs of the elderly. The elderly whose life has been extended thanks to treatment need special support for social inclusion. It should extend beyond relative "cure". Their quality of life should be addressed. It should include provision of social amenities as well. The aged are susceptible to non-communicable diseases. Their lives should be integrated into society so as to enable them access normal services and social amenities. They need jobs, gainful employment and housing. Programs should be developed and integrated into the AIDS Control Programs in order to promote the total quality of life for the elderly clients. Future HIV/AIDS programs should therefore plan for the long term post recovery needs of clients.

## 8. Community engagement

The gains should be consolidated. It is necessary to consolidate our achievements. Scaling up the test and treat strategies will significantly reduce new infections. The adolescents and young women and the youth in particular should be our priority. Broadly focus should be made on productivity especially at community and household level. Service packages and delivery platforms should be developed to respond to the social determinants of infection. Prioritize packages for which there is maximum benefit against minimum input in resources. The very significant reduction in the mother- to -child -transmission should be maintained at all costs... Engage men to stop the further spread of new infections and gender based violence. The very low level of participation by men could constrain the foreseen goals of eliminating AIDS by 2030. Let no one be left behind in realizing the goal of the elimination of HIV/AIDS by on time.

Gaps in scientific knowledge remain unanswered. We need to undertake implementation and operational research. The perfect use of scientific evidence will help sustain our achievements and improve the quality of life for all. Research should be carried out to identify the social needs of vulnerable PLWHA in respect to jobs and access to amenities including social services and recognition.

## 9. The impact of COVID

The current global COVID 19 pandemic has already impacted access to HIV/AIDS services. Since March 2020, lockdowns, curfew, travel restrictions were imposed country wide. By August 2021, about 97,000 cases and 2900 deaths were reported (Ref Standard operating procedures including social distancing limited attendance at clinics [26]. Emphasis was shifted away from HIV/AIDS to COVID 19. Occasionally there was temporary suspension of services and the fear of getting COVID from health facilities further limited access to services. According to a survey. Some 78% of the respondents reported facing challenges since the onset of COVID 19. Furthermore Coordination and central support supervision and follow up of patients was disrupted with viral load testing dropping from 96% in December 2019 to 85% in June 2021. Clinic attendance dropped by 11% in 2020 between March 2020 and June 2020. Some 5020 (0.4%) of the clients were lost and as such unable to get drug refills, and treatment noncompliance. Also ART initiation and viral load testing were reduced by 31%. CD4 testing reduced from 31–22%. There will be serious competition for both human, facility and financial resources at national and international levels. Integrating the HIV/AIDS programs may mitigate loss of funding.

Sustainability is a major is a major challenge towards "Zero cases by 2030". There will also be stiff competition for available resources. The current C OVID 19 pandemic has already impacted on health delivery and HIV/AIDS services following the lockdowns and sharing of both human and financial capacities. We need to integrate efforts at the operational levels to enhance synergy and collaboration. To undertake this approach, it is necessary to establish some national and community prevention coalitions between sectors at the community level. Uganda, for instance, has established a Community Engagement Strategy. The strategy harmonizes and integrates community efforts at village level. Family care givers provide home based care and are key members of the care team. They provide home based care, maintain community based surveillance of cases, maintain contact with clients and provide the essential supplies and advise including referrals. They make reports regularly. They, too, will respond to ethical dilemmas arising out of cultural and traditional norms. Their skills and capacity therefore should be upgraded. They should participate in community based research and evaluate interventions. All members of the community must share the burden and responsibility to change the face of HIV/AIDS. Pooled human resources will promote integration. Networks for partnerships and collaboration should be strengthened.at all levels.

## 10. Conclusion

The Abstinence- Being Faithful- Condoms strategy have effectively complemented each other and contributed to the success and reduction of HIV infection in the initial and subsequent phases of the outbreak. A decentralized community approach expanded coverage quickly and effectively. The community based strategy built bridges and solidarity among communities. The introduction of the 90–90-90 test and treat technology and the integration of behavioral and biomedical combination packages made a significant contribution to containing the HIV/AIDS pandemic. The HIV national response has been used as an entry point for the containment of other health problems including COVID 19. While there is improved longevity in general, we must also respond to the emerging social needs of the surviving elderly clients. Social programs that will assure socioeconomic inclusion for jobs, housing, and amenities are desirable for the post recovery period. Such services should be extended to include the social needs of surviving clients. Let no one be left behind as we prepare for transition to the elimination of the scourge by 2030.

## Author details

Samuel Ikwaras Okware
Uganda National Health Research Organisation, Entebbe, Uganda

*Address all correspondence to: okwares@gmail.com

## References

[1] Mbulaiteye, S., Whitworth JA,, Declinining HIV1 incidence and asssociated prevalence over 10 years in a rural population in south west Uganda: a cohort study Lancet Infectious Diseases, 2002. 360: p. 41-6.

[2] Singh S, D.J., *A, B, and C in Uganda: the roles of absitence, monogany and condom usein HIV decline*, 2003, The Allan Guttmacher Institute: Washington DC.

[3] Green E, *Rethinking AIDs prevention: learnning frm successes in developing countries*, 2003, Praeger: Westport, CT.

[4] Hogle JA, *What happened in Uganda?Declining HiV prevealence, behavior change and the national response*, 2002: Washington, DC.

[5] Project, P.H.a.n., *The ABCs' of HIV prevention. Report of a USAID technical meeting on behaviour change approaches to primary preventionof HIV/AIDS*, 2002, USAID Washington DC.

[6] Okware, S., et al., *Fighting HIV/AIDS: is success possible?* Bulletin of the World Health Organization, 2001. **79**(12): p. 1113-1120.

[7] Serwadda, D.e.a., *Slim disease, a new disease in Uganda and its association with HTLV III infection.* Lancet Infectious Diseases, 1985. **8460**: p. 849-852.

[8] Berkley, S.F., et al., *Risk factors associated with HIV infection in Uganda.* The Journal of infectious diseases, 1989. **160**(1): p. 22-30.

[9] Okware, S., et al., *Revisiting the ABC strategy: HIV prevention in Uganda in the era of antiretroviral therapy.* Postgraduate medical journal, 2005. **81**(960): p. 625-628.

[10] MoH, *STD/AIDS control program, HIV surveillance report June 2001*, in *STD/AIDS control program, HIV surveillance report*, M. J, Editor 2001, Ministry of health, AIDS Control Programme: Kampala.

[11] Berkley, S., et al., *AIDS and HIV infection in Uganda--are more women infected than men?* AIDS, 1990. **4**(12): p. 1237-1242.

[12] MoH, *Uganda population based HIV assessment(UPHIA) 2010-2017*, A. Opio, Editor 2017, MoH: Kampala.

[13] Slutkin, G., et al., *How Uganda reversed its HIV epidemic.* AIDS and behavior, 2006. **10**(4): p. 351-360.

[14] UNAIDS, *UNAIDS Strategy 2016-2021*, in *AIDSinfo (data base) updated 30 June 2020 on the track to end AIDS*2016, UNAIDS: Geneva.

[15] J, W., *Follow up HIV AIDS Cohort in Rakai, Uganda*, S. Okware, Editor 2002.

[16] UAC, *MTR of NSP 2016/2020 (Report 2019)*, in *National HIV/AIDS Strategic Plan 2020/2021-2024/2025. Leaving no one towards ending AIDS by 2030, M. Nelson*, Editor 2019, UAC: Kampala.

[17] Holmes KK, L.R., Weaver M, , *Effectiveness of condoms in preventing sexually transmitted diseases.* Bull WHO, 2004. **82**: p. 454-461.

[18] UNAIDS, *Position statement on condoms and HIV prevention*, 2004, UNAIDS UN: Geveva.

[19] MoH, *The Uganda population based HIV Impact Asseessment (UPHIA) 2010-2017.* Final report, 2019.

[20] UAC, *The Midterm Review of of the NSP 2015-2019. Final report*, 2020, UAC: Kampala

[21] UBOS, *Statistics Population Abstract, 2019*, UBOS, Editor 2019, Govenment of Uganda 01-20202019: Kampala.

[22] UBOS, *Uganda Census data,*, M.o.F.P.a.E. Development, Editor 1991, Uganda Beareau of Statistics: Kampala.

[23] UBOS, *Uganda national statistics records, 2002*, 2002, Ministry of Finance Planning and Economic Development: Kampala.

[24] UBOS, *Statistical abstract 2011*, 2011, UBOS: Kampala.

[25] UNAIDS, *Epi-data 1990-2020 AIDSinfo (database). updated 30 June 2020.*, c. AIDSinfo, Editor 2020, UNAIDS: Geneva.

[26] NSP, *National Strategic Plan 2021-2026*, UAC, Editor 2021, UAC: Kampala.

[27] Okware, S.I., *Towards a national AIDS-control program in Uganda.* The Western journal of medicine, 1987. **147**(6): p. 726-729.

[28] Muhangi, D., *Baseline study on assess to sexual and reproductive health and rights and HiV and AIDs services for LGBTI persons in Uganda. Final report of a study fo human rights awareness and promotion forum (HRAPF)*, 2018, UAC: Kampala.

[29] NAFOPHANU, *The people living with HIV Stigma Index. Uganda country assessment report*, 2019, NAFOPHANU-(The National Forum of of people living with HIV /AIDs Networks in Uganda), 2019.

[30] Semata A, *The potebntial effect of PrEP roll out on sexual risk behaviour among adolescents and young people in east ans southern Africa.*, in *unpublished* 2021.

Chapter 2

# Media Campaign Exposure and HIV/AIDS Prevention: 1980–2020

*Adamu Muhammad Hamid and Godwin Matthew Sule*

## Abstract

The interest of health communication scholars hover on relationships between HIV/AIDS message exposure and HIV knowledge, attitude and practice as the epidemic is no longer seen as only a health issue; its ramifications cover all aspects of society from economic, social structures to psychological makeup of communities. The media, under normal condition are expected to complement governments' efforts in achieving set objectives on such important issues as combating HIV/AIDS through the creation of awareness, mobilization and advocacy among other things, such as contained in the cardinal tenets of Development Media Theory. This is more so given that the only remedy to the epidemic is prevention through advocacy on the promotion of safe practices. Mass media play a central role in this direction. Exposure to HIV/AIDS messages especially on the mass media among adolescents in sub Saharan Africa has been reported as abysmal in the early 2000s, but now given growth in infrastructure and development in technology and program appeal, there emerges a need for reassessment. Given that communication particularly through the media is considered a major preventive strategy, this chapter set out to highlight a compressive review of scholarly works on HIV/AIDS media exposure, knowledge, attitudes and practices (KAP) across regions of the world, since the 80s. It is however concluded that the study of media use and HIV/AIDS KAP leaves much to be explored conceptually, methodologically and empirically.

**Keywords:** media exposure, media use, media campaigns, knowledge, attitude, practice

## 1. Introduction

The fast spread of the AIDS pandemic has engendered a vigorous debate about the role of media in fighting it. The reasons adduced, so far, are clear; that medical science has been unable to offer anything more than ways or methods of turning it from a deadly into a chronic condition, through the therapies of anti-retroviral. Because these medications are costly and complex, much emphasis and attention had shifted to prevention. This simply translates into encouraging people to change their attitudes towards the syndrome, and behaviour in that most intimate area, sex. Therefore, resources have been deployed into public information, everything from billboard campaigns to the transmission of messages about HIV/AIDS in TV programs.

> *When you are working to combat a disastrous and growing emergency, you should use every tool at your disposal. HIV/AIDS is the worst epidemic humanity has ever*

> *faced. It has spread further, faster and with more catastrophic long – term effects than any other disease. Its impact has become a devastating obstacle to development. Broadcast media have tremendous reach and influence, particularly with young people, who represent the future and who are the key to any successful fight against HIV/AIDS. We must seek to engage these powerful [media] organizations as full partners in the fight to halt HIV/AIDS through awareness, prevention and education [1]*

Substantiating the same position as early as the 90s, Hirose et al. [2] depicted a correlation between media reportage of HIV/AIDS and public risk perception of the epidemic and safer behaviour. As time went by, the complexity of the challenge raised by AIDS has become much more visible. The epidemic is no longer seen as only a health issue; its ramifications cover all aspects of society from economic, social structures to psychological makeup of communities. The pandemic has come to be recognized as a serious development issue for Third World countries since HIV/AIDS and poverty feed off each other.

In addition, as will be seen later, the social forces driving the HIV/AIDS epidemic are more clearly understood particularly through the gender dimension. Three key factors have been identified as making women or girls more vulnerable to infection: (a) the culture of silence surrounding sexuality; (b) exploitative transactional and intergenerational sex, and (c) violence against women within relationships [3]. The pandemic affects women disproportionately, not just in the prevalence of infection, but also in the impact on those affected.

The media, under normal condition are expected to complement governments' efforts in achieving set objectives on such important issues as combating HIV/AIDS through the creation of awareness, mobilization and advocacy among other things, such as contained in the cardinal tenets of Development Media Theory. This is more so given that the only remedy to the epidemic is prevention through advocacy on the promotion of safe practices. Mass media play a central role in this direction.

Combating HIV/AIDS is the number sixth item on the list of Millennium Development Goals, which signals its relative importance in the global scheme of things. Studies have passed the stage of conjecture about the epidemic at the turn of this new millennium. AIDS poses a serious challenge, which can really devastate whole regions and crack decades of national development [4]. As seen above, HIV/AIDS media exposure has been established to play a strategic central role in HIV prevention, yet literature update on the subject has been scanty, or somewhat inconsistent, sometime taking very long time gap. For strategies on HIV/AIDS risk protection to be effective, there has to be constant data updates on the trend of literature documenting advances in tracking the effect of HIV/AIDS media exposure on HIV/AIDS attitude and behavior. Policy thrust globally must rely on such evidence! This Chapter attempts to address that by documenting literature on the subject since the 80s.

In addition, Odigbo et al. [5] stated that the ability to get people's 'imagination and subsequently to change behaviours' especially in the use of the traditional media in health campaigns is yet to be captured in some of the literature. The media as game changer, through its programming has made series of attempt by providing organized agenda setting to reduce HIV/AIDS prevalence among the young adult as a means of contributing towards preventing, reducing, treatment, etc.

In spite of the important roles of communication and the only prevention or vaccine to HIV/AIDS, related literature is not definitively decisive. So it is important to keep track of scholarly contributions in the field.

For the past decades, Human Immune Deficiency Virus (HIV) or Acquired Immune Deficiency Syndrome (AIDS) has posed a lot of challenges, especially for young adultswhere HIV knowledge is limited. Media roles inthe prevention of HIV/AIDS have passed through some uncertainty as sex has not been discussed within the public sphere in most countries with high prevalence. This is as a result of objection of sex education by certain cultures and religions. Although, that does not mean that media has not been in forefront in the campaign strategies.

## 2. Media campaigns on HIV/AIDS prevention and HIV/AIDS KAP: global overview

In an extensive study, Bertrand and Anhang [6] conducted a systematic review of studies that evaluated mass media interventions in HIV/AIDS prevention, which were published between 1990 and 2004. Studies that were included in the investigation were those that evaluated mass media campaigns that had the main objective of providing information about HIV/AIDS or sexual health. And to clearly show evidence for the effectiveness of mass media intervention in HIV/AIDS prevention, the study included only studies that used a pre-intervention versus post-intervention designs, or intervention versus control design. Or an analysis of cross-sectional data comparing those who had been exposed to the media campaigns with those who had not been exposed [7].

Of the 15 programs identified by Bertrand and Anhang, 11 were from Africa, 2 from Latin America, 1 from Asia and 1 from multiple countries. One program used radio only, six used radio with supporting media, and eight others used radio and television with supporting media. Data generated and analysed by the study generally supported the effectiveness of mass media intervention to increase the knowledge of HIV/AIDS transmission modes to improve self-efficacy in condom use, to influence some social norms, to increase the amount of interpersonal communication on the subject, to increase condom use and to boost awareness of health providers. The study also found fewer significant effects for improving self-efficacy in terms of abstinence, delaying the age of first sexual experience or decreasing the number of sexual partners. Conversely, indirectly these findings would suggest weak impact in Muslim dominated countries because self-efficacy in abstinence is the most potent virtue and protection against HIV.

Specific outcomes of the study which are related to evidences that directly affected global goals on preventing HIV/AIDS among young people as outlined in the Declaration of Commitment of the UN General Assembly Special Session on AIDS are:

a. Increased awareness and knowledge of information on how to avoid HIV infection measured as

   - changes in knowledge (about modes of transmission, methods of prevention and how to tell if someone has AIDS).

b. Increased access to skills needed to avoid infection, measured as

   - self-efficacy (in abstinence, condom use).

c. Increased access to health services to avoid HIV infection, measured as

   - awareness and utilization of health products and services.

d. Decreased young people's vulnerability to HIV measured as

- more accurate perception of personal risk,
- changes in social norms (friends' approval of use of condom or abstinence).

e. Decreased HIV prevalence, measured by its proximate behavioral.

- determinants, such as
- abstinence (both intention and behavior),
- a decrease in the number of sexual partners,
- the use of condom,
- improvements in mediating factors, such as interpersonal communication (about sexual health, HIV/AIDS, condoms).

Of the nine studies examined on reporting data on knowledge of HIV transmission and prevention, four measured precisely increased knowledge of modes of HIV transmission. In Chinaaccording to the study for example, results showed significant differences, measuring both before and after interventions – in knowledge of modes of transmission, including sexual intercourse (77 percent before versus 95 percent after) sharing needles for drug use (67percent before and 95 percent after) and having multiple sex partners (69 percent before and 93 percent after). The "Tsa Banana" campaign in Botswana showed mixed results with males showing significant improvements in knowledge and females showing no significant improvements. The one study measuring knowledge of abstinence as a prevention technique, the "*HEAT*" campaign in Zambia, showed significantly higher knowledge among those who had seen the campaign as compared to those who had not (66 percent males exposed to the campaign versus 53 percent of males not exposed, 65 percent of females exposed versus 55 percent for females not exposed). In general, these studies indicated appreciable general exposure to mass media in countries including sub Saharan Africa, while Bankole et al. [8] discussed the appalling situation of media exposure among young persons in West Africa however, not the general population.

The study also found that those who had higher exposure to the Ghana Stop AIDS *Love Life* campaign were significantly more likely to believe their friends approved of delaying or avoiding sex than those with no exposure, (47 percent of females with high exposure versus 26 percent of females with no exposure). The study thus concluded that mass media programs can influence HIV related outcomes among young people, although not on every variable or in every campaign. Campaigns that included television require the highest threshold evidence, yet they also yield the strongest evidence of effects, which invariably suggested that comprehensive mass media programs are valuable. In another study on HIV/AIDS media programs in South Africa namely *Beyond Awareness II* campaign, the multimedia edutainment program *Soul City*, and the youth program *Love Life,* there was evidence of effectiveness as Coulson [9] found that the potential for mass media to reach South Africans is widely acknowledged. An estimated 99 percent of people hadaccess to radio, 75 percent had access to television and 7 percent, readership of newspapers. The finding on newspaper readership here was rather startling when compared to the high rate of literacy and relative economic viability of South Africans. More study is required here to provide insight into why the situation is low in newspaper readership in South Africa. The study also revealed sixty-nine percent of young persons watched TV five or more days a week. The study also found, prior to the development of *Soul City* (in 1997), *Beyond Awareness* campaigns (commissioned in 1995) and *Love Life* (launched in 1999), the use of the national mass media for HIV/AIDS prevention in South Africa was undeveloped. However, as a whole, the study concluded that the effective use of the mass media is a critical component of HIV/AIDS prevention.

In the Middle East, Tavoosi et al. [10] assessed the knowledge and attitudes of high school students in Iran regarding HIV/AID through a cluster sampling of 4641 students from 52 high schools in Tehran in February 2002. The results identified television as their most important source of information about AIDS. Only a few students answered all the knowledge questions correctly, which indicated low HIV knowledge among them. There were also many misconceptions about the routes of transmission- mosquito bites (33 percent) public swimming pools (21percent) and public toilets (20 percent). Forty six percent believed that HIV positive students should not be allowed to attend ordinary schools. The study also found knowledge level among the students was associated with their attitude and discipline. Since TV has been found to be a major source of information for the students on HIV/AIDS, it shows that TV programs have been ineffectual since exposure does not tally with HIV knowledge as revealed by the study.

## 3. Media role in fighting HIV/AIDS

Though journalism constitutes just a fragment of media activity, it is worth observing here the rift that has been there between the perceived role of the journalist and that of the health professional in relation to HIV/AIDS. Mcllwaine [11] states that the priorities of the journalist differ with those of health professionals: while journalists are interested in the sensational, the human-interest and dramatic angle of the subject, the health professional may deemphasize those aspects. Delineating this tension, Lupton et al. [12] referred to journalists by stating that their task is to sell their commodity i.e. news, not to serve as campaigning arm of health educators. The manner in which journalists report issues such as HIV/AIDS according to the authors can therefore 'detract from the goals of health educators'.

Apparently debunking such position however, showing the role of the journalist and that of health professional in this scenario as arriving at the same objective, Avevor [13] wrote that the role of the journalist is primarily HIV/AIDS prevention. And that they are expected to achieve that by accurate coverage of HIV/AIDS to raise public awareness and ultimately generate desired public opinion, attitude and political support, thereby tackling the syndrome by educating people. Nevertheless, the ideal role of media in combating HIV/AIDS has been aptly summarized by [1] that "education is the vaccine against HIV". The importance of HIV education is underscored by the influence of education in empowering individuals to prevent contracting the disease (The Media and HIV/AIDS: Making a difference, 2004).

Specific roles of media on the syndrome included talking about it, creating support and enabling environment for its prevention, challenging stigma and discrimination, promoting HIV/AIDS services, educating through entertainment, mainstreaming HIV/AIDS messages, emphasizing HIV/AIDS on the news agenda, and pushing leaders to act (ibid). Talking about the syndrome and creating support and enabling environment for it presuppose unlocking all channels of communication about it, thereby addressing cultural norms and confronting existing values and social norms, which are hurdles to opening up about the HIV syndrome.

Moreover, this can be achieved through education through entertainment, 'edutainment'. In Tanzania for example, it has been observed that a radio soap opera *TwendinaWakati,* meaning "let's go with the times" substantially increased the willingness of listeners to chat on the issue of HIV/AIDS [14].

In addition, recounting the limitations of their extensive study on media exposure and knowledge attitude and practice in China, Zhiwen et al. [15] and Pitts and Jackson [16] cited lack of content analyzing media output to determine the patterns of media HIV/AIDS messages as a major limitation of their study. The authors accordingly suggested complementing media and HIV/AIDS KAP studies to be complemented with content analysis of the patterns of media coverage of HIV/AIDS. The authors stated, "this study did not provide information about the nature and contents of the HIV/AIDS prevention information from these.. Content analysis studies are needed in the future to find out what kinds of such information are available through Chinese mass media sources.

Stigma and discrimination have been identified over time as driving force for the HIV epidemic; it plays the role of media to eradicate prejudice against, and encourage solidarity with people living with HIV/AIDS. Effective collaboration between the press and community organizations, government agencies and social service providers can foster for HIV/AIDS counselling, voluntary testing, care giving and treatment.To achieve optimal HIV/AIDS messaging output, media organizations needed to imbibe mainstreaming the syndrome in a number of programs, not just programs solely dedicated to it. This can be justified by the fact that the epidemic affects all facets of life. Putting the syndrome on the news agenda and encouraging leaders to act potentially create a fertile political climate for the 2030 vision of eradicating it completely. This can also be achieved by making it a news priority (in both selection and prominence).

Two decades after the emergence of HIV/AIDS, precisely in 2004, Kaisar foundation published a detailed study of press coverage of the syndrome in America conducted by [17]. After examining 9000 stories, the study concluded that, after 20 years of worlds experience with HIV/AIDS, there was a kind of 'AIDS fatigue' on the part of the US media. Journalists also reported facing difficulty in convincing their editors to run HIV/AIDS stories, partly because the syndrome has been considered just like any other disease, while far from that, actually, it is still a major cause of death in the aged 25–44 among African-Americans. In most studies on press coverage of HIV/AIDS according to [18], the common denominator was emphasis on seeking new angles and ways to convey or tell the story. A respected former journalist of Paupau New Guinea Anna Solomon observed that "AIDS is a boring report, so let's try to make it interesting" (Solomon, 2002, as cited in [19]), thereby encouraging colleagues to use imagination, sensitivity and initiative to convey the message about the syndrome.

Submissions by [17] and the veteran journalist cited above, clearly suggest that there is a growing disappearance of HIV/AIDS reports from the press as if the syndrome is no longer a serious life-threatening ailment. This situation clearly indicates the need for constant monitor of press coverage of HIV/AIDS to determine whether the situation has changed or is still looking for drastic improvement over coverage, angles, emphasis and dimensions to halt and reverse prevalence. Conversely, the news media undoubtedly served as crucial sources for the public on information about the syndrome. Seventy two percent of the United States public reported that greater part of the information they received about HIV/AIDS came from the media namely newspaper, radio and television [17]. Similarly, a national survey in India showed more than 70% of respondents indicated they received their information on HIV/AIDS from television (ibid).Evidence of press coverage of HIV/AIDS in the United States, Australia, Britain and France through the 1980s revealed a common pattern- initial slow response in terms coverage, then a heightened coverage in recognition of the emerging risk of spread and followed by a gradual fall in reportage. This is largely because of what was referred to as 'routinization' of the disease, i.e. treating it as any other health issue. These three categorizations gradually gave effect to varying degrees of sensationalism, stereotyping and complacency in coverage and proved inadequate relative to the actual scourge of the epidemic in many countries [20].

Similarly, other studies that focused on developing countries emphasized on the contents of news stories rather than frequency. Not much attention was paid to discern emerging patterns of coverage, examples are [16] in Zimbabwe, [21] in Zambia and [20] in Paupau New Guinea. A similar trend to the Western pattern of reporting was noticed though this rise-peak-decline trend was not a conscious or deliberate decision on the part of journalists or newspaper editors. In Nigeria, a study of *Daily Times of Nigeria* and the *Nigerian Tribune* released in 2008 showed slow coverage in the 90s and accelerated one in 2000s [22] though the study noticed some inconsistencies in the frequency of reports, which were higher in Februaries and Decembers, and generally lower in other months.

In a recent study, Hamid and Tamam [23] reported that the classification of the stories of HIV/AIDS in Nigerian press shows that 84% were straight news stories, 16% were feature and none was an Editorial. This dearth of interpretation reports on AIDS clearly shows that both journalists and experts had not adequately subjected the scourge of AIDS to incisive analysis. By extension, this situation further grossly limited the quantum of AIDS education and awareness in general media audience, and reflects even more, on the kind of attention the deadly epidemic received from the press in such countries. Lack of wider views, expert analysis and incisive accounts and interpretation through features and editorials may grossly affect public knowledge and attitude on HIV/AIDS. Concentrating on hard news suggests that the press, instead of acting proactively to write articles in advance, they are being reactive by waiting for events to happen before they are reported.It was also found that the news functions served by 42% of the HIV/AIDS stories are information, 42% education, 15%, awareness 8%, interpretation 12% and 23% percent advocacy as documented by the study. Scaling this finding against [24] concept of Mobilizing Information (MI), which entailed the press giving information that could be translated into meaningful health behavior or actions as key to success in combating HIV/AIDS, it could be said that the press have done fairly well by having up to 23% of stories on advocacy. After conducting an extensive research as far back as the 80s in Britain, Hamid and Tamam [23] observed that paucity of MI affected the impact of press messages. They argued that such MI communications tend to promote a particular behavior when specific details about action that can prevent health threats are explicitly given. However Cullen [25], found that editors prefer to focus on an issue rather than facilitate public participation.

In the early 90s, Osita [26] reported his study of press coverage of HIV/AIDS by four Nigerian newspapers (mostly based in southern Nigeria) in which he concluded that the press was covering the epidemic inadequately and that the reportage neglected rural areas. While [27], in a study of 3 Nigerian newspapers found that the bulk of HIV/AIDS story types were hard news and articles with no editorial. In addition, in a study of two Nigerian newspapers [28] found that HIV/AIDS stories were not emphasized on front page or given prominent placement in the pages they were carried. Similarly, Komolafe-Opadeji [22] pointed out that coverage of HIV/AIDS by Nigerian press prioritized on issues of rate of infection and workshops. And by contrast, the report of Kaisar Foundation [16] showed that 36% of all news stories on HIV/AID in the United States press was on educating people how to protect themselves.

The Panos Institute extensively studied newspaper coverage of HIV/AIDS in the region worst hit by the epidemic, southern African countries. The study was conducted in eight countries of the region: Zambia, Zimbabwe, Namibia, Lesotho, South Africa, Botswana, Swaziland and Malawi in 2003. In the study, tremendous improvement on coverage was noticed in the 80s and then stories gradually became sensational and insensitive to those affected by the HIV/AIDS epidemic. In the 90s, such military metaphors as 'killer disease' 'HIV/AIDS victims" gave way to a more humane and sensitive expressions as 'people living with AIDS', and gradually HIV/AIDS news report was seen as development story which educates people and gives hope rather than just a health story [29]. That period witnessed more stories of hope rather than illustrations of despair with pictures of emaciated people and scary statistics gradually became less preponderant (ibid). Majority of news reports were also noticed to be about workshops, speeches and conferences just as happened in the West as reported by [16]. Panos Institute [29] concluded, the corpus of HIV/AIDS reports omitted the voices of those affected and became 'monotonous and less appealing to readers.'

In a related study also, Jing [30] tested relationships between the coverage of HIV/AIDS news frames or themes and how the different themes were emphasized in the US and Chinese newspapers and found a significant relationship between HIV/AIDS story frames and their emphasis in the newspapers studied. Similarly, discussing the analytic procedures of newspaper content analysis, Panos Institute [29] showed that newspaper content variables sometimes have statistical relationships with one another. They elucidated for example, that newspaper stories' sources mostly have relationship with their geographic focuses. Though much interesting in revealing patterns of newspaper coverage, extremely few newspaper content analysis paid attention to testing relationships between content variables. Such studies mostly focus on only descriptive statistics.

## 4. Knowledge of HIV/AIDS and attitude change

Knowledge of HIV/AIDS is closely linked to people's consciousness on avoiding the disease. An extensive study on knowledge and consciousness was conducted on "self – awareness" by [30] which posits that each one formulates body of personal knowledge about one's characteristics. In his view, self-awareness has significant influence on behavior, adding that we can scarcely have consistent and favorable attitudes and beliefs towards ideas which we have not previously encountered.

In instances, knowledge level of HIV/AIDS is predicted by socio-economic status. In a study conducted in Lebanon, education and income were found to be significantly related to knowledge of HIV transmission and prevention among women. In terms of income, women in richest quintile were found to be 4 times more likely to be knowledgeable than women in the poverty quintile. Almost half applies to women with the highest education as compared to women with elementary education or less than that [31].

In an earlier study, Lynch and Peer [32] reports that a study by UNFPA stated that sexually transmitted infection (STIs) are generally major public health challenges that have received public health attention in the two decades before the study because of their serious social and economic consequences. Knowledge of STIs according to the study is important because of associated disabilities and more importantly because of the "close association between STIs and HIV/AIDS and how they could be contacted and prevented."

In this key area of HIV/AIDS knowledge, it is worth highlighting that the area of study – Northeast Nigeria-- is remarkably weak in terms of HIV and STIs knowledge especially among the female population. For example, way back since 2004, UNFPA [33] also showed that only 7.7% of the female populations in Bauchi have STIs complete knowledge according to recognized indicators. The female figure in Gombe is 23.0%, in Borno 26.0%, in Katsina 25.7% and in Kebbi 18.7%. And in all the states, the investigation showed that HIV awareness is relatively lower among the female population. Recent data on this key index of HIV prevention appears to be lacking.

A potent measure in increasing HIV/AIDS knowledge is educational program in mass media. In a study conducted on YARD (Young Adults Reproductive Health) program, Kirby (1999) as cited in [34] reviewed the evidence on the effectiveness of the program in the United States, and the work suggested that HIV/AIDS education efforts are more effective than the general reproductive health education programs, possibly because they are more successful in attracting the attention of boys.

Bankole (2004) as cited in [34], states that despite the international attention that the HIV/AIDS epidemics has received, knowledge of the disease is not usual among adolescents. Perceptions of personal risk are sometimes at odds with reality. According to him, while at least 90% of the women and men aged 15–19 years in most countries in sub-Saharan Africa have heard of HIV/AIDS, substantial proportion in some countries have not; 43% - 46% of young women in Chad and Niger, 26% in Nigeria and 19–21% in Burkina Faso. In majority of countries with available data, half of adolescent women who have heard of HIV/AIDS think they are at risk of becoming infected. But in Ghana, Nigeria, Niger and Tanzania, no more than three in 10 young women consider themselves at risk. Adolescents' perception of risk is not always consistent with HIV prevalence in different countries. In Kenya, Cameron, and Zambia for example, only about half of young women and men who have heard of HIV/AIDS think they are at risk, even though prevalence is high in these countries. On the other hand, in Mozambique, another country with high prevalence about 7 in 10 adolescent women and men who have heard of HIV/AIDS believe that they are at risk.

According to [35] awareness of HIV/AIDS is generally high in both urban and rural areas in Nigeria and between males and females of all age groups though in north east and north central zones, 2 out of 10 respondents in the survey have never heard of HIV/AIDS. Knowledge about HIV/AIDS prevention and transmission routes is fair with 59% (63% males and 56% females) knowing all the four main transmission routes: Sexual intercourse, blood transfusion, mother – to – child and sharing of sharp objects. The survey went further to reveal that misconceptions about HIV transmission are still high. Twenty five per cent of females and 21% of males believed HIV is transmitted through sharing of toilets. As far as prevention is concerned, only 51% (42% of female and 60% of males) reports that one can reduce the risk of contracting HIV by being faithful to uninfected partner. Six out of 10 respondents know that healthy looking person can be HIV positive. On mother to child transmission, 65% of females and 71% of males know that HIV can be transmitted during pregnancy.

Federal Ministry of Health [35] also indicates that the awareness of AIDS in Nigeria is higher among men than women with 97% of men and 80% of women reporting that they have heard of AIDS. The survey showed no significant differences in knowledge among men by background social and demographic characteristics. However, there are significant differences among women living in households ranked lowest on prosperity index (70%). Even though there is sometimes an appreciable level of HIV knowledge among respondents, however, misconceptions about the disease hamper progress in communication efforts to stem its prevalence (Soyombo, 2005 as cited in [32]).

Expounding on the correlation between media exposure and HIV/AIDS knowledge, a study of media use and HIV/AIDS knowledge in northwestern Ethiopia by

[36] delivered mixed results. Exploring the knowledge gap resulting from mass media use disparities in the study population, precisely checking the relationship between mass media exposure relating to HIV/AIDS and HIV/AIDS knowledge, the study found that in the total population of the respondents mass media exposure is not a significant predictor of knowledge related to HIV/AIDS. But at the same time however, the study showed that there is a negative relationship in knowledge gap between respondents with high education and those with low education as HIV/AIDS media use increases. Put differently, the knowledge gap between the two groups closes with the increase in HIV/AIDS media consumption. Therefore in this study, the impact path from media exposure to HIV/AIDS safe practice is hypothesized to be mediated by HIV/AIDS knowledge because in the study above, though faintly, a relationship is figured out between media use and HIV/AIDS knowledge. This study will clarify further, such a relationship.

Much has been written about the linkage between HIV knowledge and attitude change, but from the standpoint of psychology, knowledge about an idea is often quite different from using it. Most individuals know about many innovations, many of which they do not adapt to. Here, the reason could be the individual does not regard the idea as relevant to his/her situation. Buttressing this relationship of knowledge and attitude change, Ajzen and Fishbein [37] posited that attitude is typically viewed as a latent variable that is assumed to guide or influence behavior.

In a research on sexual behavior and perception of AIDS in Benin City, Evelyn and Osafor (1990) as cited in [34], revealed that despite good HIV/AIDS knowledge, a high percentage of the study sample admitted having multiple sex partners with only a negligible proportion using condom. This shows a risky behavior against the knowledge about HIV prevention.Dependingon the nature of a particular society, a range of issues are raised about the use of condom. For example, based on an assessment of HIV/AIDS among youth and adult men with steady sex partners in four states of Nigeria, condom use depends on one's perception of and desire for the trust of their partner(s). Introducing the use of condom in a relationship is in some cases seen as evidence of, or suspicion of infidelity among sex partners. Reference to "skin – to – skin" contact among the majority of sex workers' clients as well as other men and youth with multiple partners placed groups at a heightened risk of contracting HIV [38].

## 5. Conclusion

Based on the review, it is concluded that media exposure is a necessary but not a sufficient precursor for HIV/AIDS safe behaviour and attitude. Media exposure reinforces other components of HIV/AIDS knowledge and perhaps, interpersonal discussions on HIV/AIDS vide media agenda setting to affect HIV/AIDS favourable attitude and safe practice.

In spite of well acknowledged potential of mass media in HIV prevention, little is known in terms of the knowledge gap on HIV/AIDS that exists in societies as a result of disparities in media exposure and the concomitant effect of HIV/AIDS media use on attitude and behaviour regarding HIV/AIDS. This study is a response to such paucity in literature. It is also concluded that fusing HIV/AIDS-related information can narrow the gap in HIV/AIDS knowledge in a given social milieu, and as well address the challenges of negative HIV/AIDS attitudes and risky practice. From the evidence garnered in this study it is further concluded that the propositions of media Accumulation theory and Klapper's (1964) reinforcement perspectives gained much support thereby rendering the arguments of the critics of the transmission model of HIV/AIDS preventive media campaign theories implausible and very weak, as cited in [39]. Prolonged periods of persistent supply of HIV/AIDS preventive campaigns on condom use has the capacity to alter the long engendered negative view of condoms in North-eastern Nigerian societies. So Western developed HIV/AIDS preventive campaigns based on social psychology do have success.

The mass media remain a major source of HIV/AIDS information for majority of adolescents girls in North-eastern Nigeria and West Africa in general and Hausa Home Video provides a potentially big window for mass media access to and addressing adolescents on HIV/AIDS. In line with the improvements in literacy and media exposure among adolescents however, the press needed to pay more attention to HIV/AIDS protective or preventive stories instead of overemphasis on care for people living with HIV/AIDS which is a reactionary approach.

Though there was a remarkable improvement noticed in this study in terms of the scope of HIV/AIDS coverage by the press as compared to the findings of previous studies in Africa and elsewhere, the press are not doing enough by not making the HIV/AIDS stories prominent on front pages or in back pages or dedicating an editorial to it or even illustrating the stories with attention catching design devices. At least when the emphasis the press give to the subject is compared to the fact Africa is the bearer of the largest HIV/AIDS burden.

## 6. Recommendation

Based on the findings in this study, it is hereby suggested that strategy must be adopted in HIV/AIDS media messages conceptualization process to emphasize messages that advancethe knowledge of adolescents on HIV/AIDS specific issues of prevention, transmission, demography and epidemiology and deemphasize those that directly instruct them to change behavior. This is largely because this study establishes that HIV/AIDS message exposure only affects HIV/AIDS behavior through HIV/AIDS knowledge. By improving adolescents HIV/AIDS knowledge reservoir, this study contends, behavior change is almost guaranteed. Put differently, this study supports designing programs aimed at directly influencing HIV/AIDS knowledge among adolescents, thereby subliminally targeting attitude and behavior change. For example, the media can emphasize on issue-specific knowledge on HIV risky practices, and the knowledge that the practice is risky could perhaps motivate behavior change.

HIV/AIDS messages producers and reporters must research the interpretations of target audiences of such messages before any media campaign slogans are released. If possible misinterpretations are not controlled, the campaign messages are less likely to reap the desirable impact. While the ABC and safe sex campaigns can be suggested by this study to continue, findings also indicate that mother-to-child transmission and multiple sex partner slogans are prone to negative interpretations and they are suggested to stop and be replaced by other phraseology that are less prone to misinterpretation. Again, HIV/AIDS campaign producers and news reporters should consider campaigns that extol the virtue in virginity and similar themes like eschewing nudity or wearing sexually provocative dress in Northeast Nigeria because they are in consonance with Islamic philosophy on chastity and other praise-worthy values that are deterrent to HIV/AIDS risky practices.

The press in Nigeria should emphasize stories on the risks of HIV/AIDS and publish adequate editorials and features with Mobilizing Information in order to help the public to translate such information into meaningful health actions. Newspaper reporting on HIV/AIDS should also avoid over concentrating in the urban centres; serious effort should be made to reveal the overall comprehensive outlook of the HIV situation down to the grassroots. Newspapers should employ designate professional health reporters as that will increase frequency of HIV/AIDS features and encourage the newspapers to have editorials with informed opinions and official stand over issues concerning HIV/AIDS. Editorial design and production of newspapers should pay close attention in page layout by emphasizing HIV/AIDS stories on the upper left quadrant of pages, accompanying the stories with attention capturing devices such as color, picture and cartoon and most importantly by accentuating the stories on front pages.

## Author details

Adamu Muhammad Hamid* and Godwin Matthew Sule
Department of Mass Communication, The Federal Polytechnic, Bauchi, Nigeria

*Address all correspondence to: hamidadam00@gmail.com

## References

[1] UNAIDS, (2004). *Media and HIV/AIDS: Making the Difference.* Retrieved from http://data.unaids.org/publications/irc-pub06/jc1000-media_en.pdf

[2] Hirose, H., Nakaune, N., Ishizuka, T., Tsuchida, S., & Takanashi, Y. (1998). A study on the role of AIDS mass communication: How do the mass media affect HIV testing behavior?. Japanese psychological research, *40*(4), 246-255.

[3] Krüger, F. (2005). Ethical journalism in a time of AIDS. African Journal of AIDS Research, *4*(2), 125-133.

[4] Ugande, G.B. (2007). Radio Benue and HIV/AIDS awareness creation in Vandiekya local government area of Benue State: An Evaluation. A Paper presented at ACCE Conference, Zaria 2007.

[5] Odigbo, B., UgwuOgbu, S., & Ekemezie, L. I. (2017). Effect of Mass Media and Africa Traditional Media on HIV/Aids Prevention Social Marketing Campaigns in Nigeria. *International Review of Management and Business Research,* 6(2), 462-471.1

[6] Bertrand, J. T., & Anhang, R. (2006). The effectiveness of mass media in changing HIV/AIDS-related behaviour among young people in developing countries. Technical Report Series-World Health Organization, *938*, 205.

[7] Bertrand, J. T. & Anhang, R. (2006). "The effectiveness of Mass Media in Changing HIV/AIDS Prevention at Young People in Developing Countries" in Ross, D.A., Dick, B. & Ferguson J.(eds) (2006) *Preventing HIV/AIDS in Young People: a Systematic Review of Evidence From Developing Countries*: World Health organization

[8] Bankole, A., Singh, S., Woog, V., & Wulf, D. (2004). *Risk and protection: youth and HIV/AIDS in sub-Saharan Africa.* New York: The Guttmacher Institute.

[9] Coulson, N. (2002). *Developments in the use of the mass media at the national level for HIV/AIDS prevention in South Africa. The Communication Initiative.* (Publishers not identified)

[10] Tavoosi, A., Zaferani, A., Enzevaei, A., Tajik, P., & Ahmadinezhad, Z. (2004). Knowledge and attitude towards HIV/AIDS among Iranian students. BMC Public Health, *4*(1), 4-17 https://doi.org/10.1186/1471-2458-4-17

[11] Mcllwaine, S. (2001). Science and journalism: A Mexican stand-off? Australian Journalism Review, 23 (2), 167-188.

[12] Lupton, D., Chapman, S., & Wong, W. (1993). Back to complacency: AIDS in the Australian press. Health Education Research, 8 (1), 5-17.

[13] Avevor, D. (2013). HIV and AIDS reporting: The Role of the journalist. Retrieved from https://www.modernghana.com/.../hiv-and-aids-reporting-the-role-of-the-journalist.html

[14] Peterson, J. L., & DiClemente, R. J. (Eds.). (2000). *Handbook of HIV prevention*. Taylor

[15] Zhiwen, X., Xiaoming, L., Danhua, L., & Cheuk, C. T. (2015) Mass Media and HIV/AIDS Prevention Among Female Sex Workers in Beijing, China

[16] Pitts, M., & Jackson, H. (1993). Press coverage of AIDS in Zimbabwe: A five year plan. AIDS Care, 5 (2), 223-30.

[17] Brodie, M., Hamel, E., Brady, L. A., Kates, J., & Altman, D. E. (2004). AIDS at 21: Media coverage of the

HIV epidemic 1981-2002. Columbia Journalism Review, *42*(6), A1.

[18] Cullen, T. (2003). *HIV/AIDS: 20 years of press coverage*. Western Australia: ECU Publications.

[19] Cullen, T. (2006). *HIV/AIDS: 25 years of press coverage*. Western Australia: ECU Publications.

[20] Cullen, T. A. (2011). Health reporting: The missing links. ejournalist, 11(2), 137-148. Original article available at http://ro.ecu.edu.au/ecuworks2011/47

[21] Kasoma, F. P., Kwame Boafo, S. T., & Arnoldo, C. A. (2000). The Zambian newspapers and AIDS. Media and HIV/AIDS in East and Southern Africa: A Resource Book. Paris, UNESCO.

[22] Komolafe-Opadeji, H. O. (2008). Promoting public awareness of HIV/AIDS in Africa: Follow-up to a pilot study. Library Philosophy and Practice. Retrieved from http://digitalcommons.unl.edu/libphilprac/194

[23] Hamid, A. M. & Tamam, E. T. (2018) Press Coverage of HIV/AIDS in Northern Nigeria: A Study of *Daily Trust* Newspaper. Human Communication, 1(1), 106-126

[24] Kristiansen, C. and Harding C., (1984). Mobilization of health behavior by the press in Britain. Journalism Quarterly 61 (2): 364-370.

[25] Cullen, T. (2000). *Repeating mistakes: press coverage of HIV/AIDS in Papua New Guinea and the South Pacific* (A Doctoral dissertation), University of Queensland.

[26] Osita, N. C. (1993) Press coverage of the Acquired Immunodeficiency Syndrome (AIDS) in Nigeria: A Content analytic study. (A Master's thesis submitted to the Department of Mass Communication University of Nigeria, Nsukka).

[27] Anim, E. (2011). The Perception of the HIV and AIDS Pandemic by the Nigerian Press. Journal of Communication, 2(2), 105-116.

[28] Odoemelam, L., Onumadu, F., & Arua, I. (2008) Media coverage of hiv/aids: a content analysis of two Nigerian newspapers (The Guardian and Daily Sun). Education, *26*(18), 18-18.

[29] Panos Institute (2004). *Lessons for today and tomorrow: An analysis of HIV reporting in Southern Africa*. Lusaka: Panos Southern Africa.

[30] Jing, T. (2006). Framing AIDS: A comparative analysis of AIDS coverage in US and Chinese Newspaper, 2001-2004. Perspectives: Working papers in English and Communication, *17*(1), 1-21.

[31] Kobeissi, L., El Kak, F. H., Khawaja, M., & Khoshnood, K. (2015). HIV/AIDS-Related Knowledge and Its Association With Socioeconomic Status Among Women: Results of Lebanese Survey for Family Health (PAPFAM) 2004. Asia-Pacific Journal of Public Health, *27*(2), NP734–NP745. http://doi.org/10.1177/1010539511431299

[32] Lynch, S. & Peer, L. (2002). Analyzing newspaper content a how–to guide: Including national comparison data for US daily newspapers. Readership Institute, Northwestern University. Retrieved from http://www.orau.gov/cdcynergy/erc/Content/activeinformation/resources/NewspaperContentAnalysis.pdf

[33] UNFPA (2004). *Reproductive Health and Gender Indicators, Baseline Survey of Assisted States in Nigeria*. Author

[34] Abubakar, A. (2006). HIV/AIDS and community behavior in Ningi, Bauchi State. (A Degree

project submitted to the Department Mass Communication, University of Maiduguri, Nigeria).

[35] Federal Ministry of Health (2003) *Nigeria Demographic and Health Survey (2003)*.Author

[36] Bekalu, M. A., & Eggermont, S. (2013). Media use and HIV/AIDS knowledge: a knowledge gap perspective. Health Promotion International, *29*(4), 739-750.

[37] Ajzen, I & Fishbein, M. (1975). *Belief, attitude, intention and behavior: An Introduction to theory and Research* MA: Addison – Wesley.

[38] GrundfestSchoepf, B. (2003). Uganda: lessons for AIDS control in Africa. Review of African Political Economy, *30*(98), 553-572.

[39] Airhihenbuwa, C.O. & Obregon, R.(2000). A Critical analysis of Theories/ of Models Used in Health Communication for HIV/AIDS in Journal *Health communication,* vol 5: pp 5-15

Chapter 3

# Prevention of HIV Perinatal Transmission: The Role of Sexual and Reproductive Health Services for Women Living with HIV

*Marcela Gómez-Suárez*

## Abstract

With the evolution in prevention, diagnosis, and treatment of HIV/AIDS, ending the infection as a public health threat worldwide has become a real possibility included within the United Nations Sustainable Development Goal Project 2030. However, some countries and even entire regions are not on track to reach this target due to increased new infections in young populations. Young women (15–24 years) represent 48% of the new HIV cases globally. Research shows these women have significant unmet sexual and reproductive health (SRH) needs, with high rates of unplanned pregnancies, increased HIV perinatal transmission (HIV-PT) risk, and higher maternal morbidity and mortality. Granting access to SRH services based on rights for women living with HIV is a cost-effective alternative to reducing new infections in children by promoting respect for women's reproductive options. This chapter addresses the role of SRH services based on rights for women living with HIV within HIV-PT. It also summarizes the new "Consolidated Guideline on Sexual and Reproductive Health and Rights of Women Living with HIV"; designed by the World Health Organization as a global recommendation for SRH programs and services that promote gender equality and human rights for women living with HIV.

**Keywords:** HIV, AIDS, perinatal HIV transmission, vertical HIV transmission, unplanned pregnancies, sexual and reproductive health, access to health services, women's health, women's rights

## 1. Introduction

In the last decades, the HIV/AIDS picture has changed notably with global health policy accomplishments for prevention, diagnosis, treatment, and follow-up, improving people's quality of life and turning the overwhelming prognosis of a fatal disease into a chronic, treatable condition. The progress in the control of HIV/AIDS has stimulated a debate on the possibility of ending it as a public health threat by 2030, and it has become a substantial element of the United Nations third Sustainable Development Goal Project 2030 (SDG-3.3). The goal is to decline new HIV infections and AIDS-related deaths by 90% between 2010 and 2030 [1].

 IntechOpen

Despite all the public health advances related to HIV, there are countries and even entire regions that are not on track to reach the global target due to new infections. In 2019 the Joint United Nations Program on HIV/AIDS (UNAIDS) reported 1.7 million people with newly acquired HIV infections. Eastern Europe and Central Asia registered a 72% rise in new HIV infections since 2010. New HIV infections have also risen in the Middle East and North Africa by 22% and 21% in Latin America. Certain regions like Eastern and Southern Africa are exceptions to these rates, with a sustained 38% reduction in new infections since 2010 [2].

A third of new HIV infections affect young populations. With the change in transmission trends during the past two decades, more women have become infected by sexual transmission within high-risk partners. They currently represent more than half of the people living with HIV worldwide and 48% of the new cases reported each year. Health risks for acquiring HIV infection are especially acute for adolescent girls and young women aged 15–24 years, and AIDS persists as the fourth leading cause of death in middle and low-income countries [3]. The risk for acquiring HIV, especially in young women and adolescent girls, arises from multiple reasons, including unfavorable health social determinants such as economic dependence; poverty; lack of education and formal work opportunities; adolescent marriage; intrafamily and institutional violence, and limited access to Sexual and Reproductive Health Services based on Rights (SRHSR) like family planning and adolescent-friendly health services among others [4].

Women living with HIV (WLHIV) have significant unmet sexual, and reproductive health (SRH) needs leading to high rates of unplanned pregnancies. Research shows that these necessities are even three times higher than women without HIV and increase the number of new HIV infections in their children due to HIV perinatal transmission (HIV-PT); and higher maternal morbidity and mortality. Studies also show that these unmet needs increase the number of unsafe abortions and unwanted sterilizations, due to health providers and patient's misinformation about HIV and pregnancy [5, 6].

To accomplish the SDG-3, the elimination of HIV-PT is a must. Globally, in 2019, 1.8 million children were living with HIV, with 95,000 AIDS-related deaths and 150,000 new infections. Even though new HIV infections among children have declined by 52% since 2010, some countries, especially in concentrated epidemic settings, have maintained stationary HIV-PT rates for the past ten years, far away from the elimination goals. HIV-PT is still considered a public health problem representing the impossibility of health systems to end a preventable disease with immense repercussions for children's lives, families, and the community [7]. In HIV-positive populations, studies have shown a close relationship between women's SRH and HIV-PT prevention. Granting access to SRHSR for WLHIV is a cost-effective alternative to reducing new infections in children by promoting planned and desired pregnancies and promoting respect for WLHIV's reproductive options as part of the United Nations International covenant on rights [8].

The present chapter addresses the relevance of SRHSR for WLHIV within HIV-PT reduction. The first part explores aspects of women's vulnerability to acquire and live with HIV and the relationship of these determinants with SRH. The final part summarizes the 2017 World Health Organization's (WHO) "Consolidated Guideline on Sexual and Reproductive Health and Rights of Women Living with HIV," related to the HIV-PT prevention recommendations based on rights [9].

*DOI: http://dx.doi.org/10.5772/intechopen.98306*

## 2. Women and HIV

An estimated 20.1 million women were living with HIV worldwide at the end of 2020, representing approximately 55% of all HIV infections [10, 11]. Also, almost half of the estimated 1.7 million new HIV infections in adults for the same year globally were among women. HIV infection remains the leading cause of death among women of reproductive age [12]. Most women acquire HIV through heterosexual relations with high-risk partners. In sub-Saharan Africa, 59% of people with HIV are those, and those aged 15 to 24 years are eight times more likely than their male peers to be infected [13]. In the Caribbean, young women are twice as likely to be infected as men. In Eastern Europe and Central Asia, injecting drug use (IDU) and sex work are the primary drivers of the epidemic. One-third of women acquired HIV infection by injecting drugs, and 50% from partners who inject drugs. Latin America's epidemic concentrates among men who have sex with men (MSM), but more than 20% of the region's MSM also report having sex with women [14, 15].

### 2.1 Risk factors for HIV acquisition in women

Women have differential vulnerabilities to HIV acquisition studied in different contexts. Below are some of the core biological, behavioral, and social determinants risk factors related to the heterosexual transmission that individually and synergistically contribute to these HIV infection rates among women globally.

#### *2.1.1 Biological risk factors*

Research has presented evidence about the relationship between the female reproductive tract, the immune system inflammatory response, and the vaginal microbiome, decreasing or increasing women's vulnerability to HIV infection. Interestingly, there is a unique balance between the female mucosal immune system and the hormonal system at the cellular level. This balance intends to protect women from genital infection while permitting an embryo's survival [16–18].

Genital tract inflammation (infection, microscopic abrasions that result from sexual activity, douching, or other causes) also increases women's susceptibility to HIV infection [19]. Different studies demonstrate the importance of the vaginal microbiome in maintaining the acidic environment that protects against HIV and suggests that lower genital tract infections can promote HIV acquisition among women [20, 21].

#### *2.1.2 Behavioral risk factors*

The risk of heterosexual acquisition of HIV varies from as low as one per 1000 contacts between uninfected and infected individuals to one transmission per three contacts. Factors including male circumcision status, HIV viral load concentration; sexually transmitted infections; alterations of vaginal flora, and anal intercourse increase women's risk and contribute to the variation in these estimates of transmission. Factors such as hormonal contraception may also affect HIV acquisition risk. Sexual partners' participation in concurrent sexual relationships, especially MSM, and age disparity with intergenerational relationships between young women and older men, increase individual women's risk of acquiring infection and help spread HIV throughout the population [22–25].

Sexual violence represents a significant risk for HIV infection acquisition among women [26, 27]. In HIV prevalent settings, women who experience intimate partner violence are 50% more likely to acquire HIV than women who do not have these experiences. In medium and low-income settings, gender-based violence is common for women and increases their risk for HIV acquisition. This risk is related to genital injury due to forced intercourse with an infected partner, limitations to negotiate safer sexual behaviors, and patterns of sexual risk-taking among women who experienced abuse during childhood or adolescence. War, migration, displacement, and conflict situations also increase women's risk of experiencing sexual violence, including rape and HIV acquisition [28, 29].

#### *2.1.3 Social determinants of health as risk factors*

Research shows how women's HIV risk acquisition is consistently associated with disadvantageous economic security, education, and other structural determinants prevalent in medium and low-income settings. A systematic literature review from eighteen countries performed in Latin America showed that most women who became HIV infected were young, less-educated, working in informal jobs, and users of public health services. Besides the structural health determinants related to HIV, these women also faced barriers to accessing contraceptive alternatives and SRHSR imposing a limit to their capacity to make autonomous reproductive decisions [30, 31]. Gender inequality is an essential structural factor underlying usual risk factors associated with HIV acquisition. Women's unequal educational, social, economic, and political status represents an inherent disadvantage; unequal power limits their ability to negotiate at a relationship and family level. Also, there is a high prevalence of violence, and women who experience trauma, abuse, or other forms of sexual violence are at increased risk for HIV acquisition [32].

#### *2.1.4 Differential HIV acquisition risks in young women*

The standard definition of young women includes all those falling within the ages of 15–24 years. Between these ages, young women undergo significant transitions in lifestyle, maturity, and legal rights, which place them at different vulnerabilities for HIV acquisition. Young women are more susceptible to HIV infection than older women. Some biological factors may explain this age-variability in vulnerability. For example, the immature cervix has a more significant proportion of genital mucosa exposed to HIV, highly susceptible to infection. They also have relatively high levels of genital inflammation, which have consistently been reported to increase HIV acquisition risk [32, 33].

Vulnerabilities in youth often are incremented by the interaction of the effects of social disparities and sexual behaviors. Choosing a sexual partner, early sexual debut, teen pregnancies; early school dropout; and sexual violence increase adolescent girls and young women's vulnerability to acquiring HIV infection and maintain them in cycles of poverty and dependency. Young women, on average, have their first sexual encounters during their teenage years: in sub-Saharan Africa and Latin America, about 60% of young women are sexually active by the time they reach the age of 18. However, unprotected sex between adolescents can result in pregnancy, HIV transmission is not frequent. In contrast, sex with an older man is more likely to result in HIV acquisition and pregnancy. Data show that women who start their sexual life at a young age have an older first sexual partner and have experienced sexual coercion [33–35].

## 3. Living with HIV

WLHIV must face complex lives with profound physical and psychological consequences. HIV/AIDS represents a dangerous triangle as these women must meet their condition in different roles, as a patient, as a mother, and as a carer of partners, parents, or orphans with AIDS. In middle and low-income settings, WLHIV also live painful lives of exclusion. They are rejected by their family, friends, and partners. With low access to education and work possibilities, thousands have lost their lives, and many more have been unable to fulfill them [35–37].

Since it was first identified, HIV has been linked with some kind of "sexual misbehavior," contributing to the high level of stigma and discrimination associated with the infection [38]. Women are often more susceptible to the stigma related to HIV and are frequently referred to as "transmitters" [39, 40]. Discrimination discourages them from seeking the vital medical and psychological care they need during the illness. HIV stigma in women is associated with feelings of uncertainty and loss, low self-esteem, fear, anxiety, depression, and even suicidal ideation [41–43].

Different systematic reviews have examined stigma and discrimination in WLHIV, revealing the constant fear related to their medical condition and the painful effects of stigmatization and discrimination, including social rejection, denial, even violence within family and community. The rejection and discrimination extends to institutional violence by health care professionals. These studies also highlight that women face higher levels of discrimination from society just because they are women [43–45].

### 3.1 Sexual and reproductive health in WLHIV

According to the United Nations Population Fund (UNPFA), SRH implies that people can have a satisfying and safe sex life, the capability to reproduce, and the freedom to decide if, when, and how often to do so. There are essential links between HIV/AIDS and women's SRH. For many, HIV represents the most challenging SRH issue; frequently diagnosed during pregnancy, HIV infection in women arises the necessity to cope with many fears and uncertainties related to SRH like death, guilt, side-effects from treatment, pregnancy, and delivery complications, HIV-PT, childbearing, and breastfeeding [46]. WLHIV have a high risk for unplanned pregnancies, reported as three times higher than in women without HIV. The consequences of unplanned pregnancies can be profound, placing WLHIV at greater risk of death during the pregnancy and postpartum period and leading to lower antiretroviral therapy (ART), adherence and higher attrition rates in prenatal care, and higher risk for HIV-PT [47].

One of the most basic SRH interventions is family planning, an important HIV prevention strategy for women. For WLHIV, contraceptive counseling is recommended by UNAIDS to prevent HIV-PT, advocating for planned and desired pregnancies and avoiding unplanned pregnancies. WLHIV who want and plan their pregnancies have better treatment adherence and lower risk of perinatal transmission and complications [48].

Barriers to access SRH represent a lost opportunity for HIV prevention, follow-up, and counseling. A lack of comprehensive SRHSR means that women cannot take care of their SRH rights and increases the risk of HIV infection or HIV-PT due to unplanned pregnancies. Studies show that barriers to access SRH services take many forms, including denial of access to services, non-integrated services implying different appointments for HIV and SRH, discrimination and institutional violence from service providers, and poor-quality services [49].

Within some settings, procedures related to SRH still are performed without consent, including sterilization and abortion. These interventions also deter women from accessing services and are usually associated with complicated relationships with healthcare providers who do not fully understand childbirth and HIV laws and misinterpret information about HIV-PT preventive measures during pregnancy, delivery, and postpartum [50, 51]. Gender-based violence acts as an important barrier to the uptake of HIV testing and counseling, to the disclosure of HIV-positive status, and antiretroviral treatment (ART) uptake and adherence. Fear and violence lead women to avoid disclosing their HIV status, causing them to miss medical appointments and lose HIV care and follow-up [52, 53].

## 4. Sexual and Reproductive Health based on Rights (SRHR), a guideline for WLHIV

WLHIV do not have equitable access to quality health services in some settings and face multiple forms of stigma and discrimination. They are disproportionately vulnerable to violence, including violations of their sexual and reproductive rights [6, 7]. In 2017, the WHO, in response to requests from different organizations worldwide, and seeking to bring together new and existing recommendations and good practice statements related to the SRHR of WLHIV into one document, developed the new "Consolidated Guideline on Sexual and Reproductive Health and Rights of Women Living with HIV." This effort was meant to help countries plan, develop and monitor programs and services promoting gender equality and human rights acceptable and appropriate for women living with HIV [9].

The consolidated guideline advocates for a comprehensive, woman-centered approach to SRHR, from women's perspectives, their families, and communities. This approach maintains the guiding principles of gender equality and human rights. The base for developing this WHO guideline was a global survey conducted to assess the SRHR of WLHIV to prioritize their values and preferences. The survey is the largest performed to date and included 945 WLHIV from 94 countries [54]. The starting point of the guide is where a woman knows her HIV diagnosis. From there, it covers critical issues for providing SRHR-related services to support more effective health interventions and better health outcomes.

The guideline addresses new evidence-based good practice statements establishing the close relationship between SRHR and HIV within the framework represented in **Figure 1**. The core is grounded in a woman-centered approach (pink circle), the enabling environment strategies (outer purple circle), and the health interventions needed (central blue segments).

A woman-centered approach to access health services involves considering WLHIV as active participants and beneficiaries of good-quality, efficient, and reliable health systems capable of responding to their needs, rights, and preferences. They are also meant to promote gender equality and women empowerment for decision-making as the core for the achievement of SRHR.

The enabling environment strategies for WLHIV encompass eight activities to assist them in overcoming service uptake barriers, stimulate SRHSR use, and encourage continued engagement: promotion of healthy sexuality across the life course, from adolescence to menopause, with SRHR and HIV programs to meet women's health priorities in all epidemic contexts, including psychosocial support interventions, such as support groups and peer support [55]; facilitation of economic empowerment and resource access to reduce WLHIV inherent vulnerabilities; integration of SRHSR and HIV services to increase access to and improve retention in care and services; protection from intrafamily and institutional

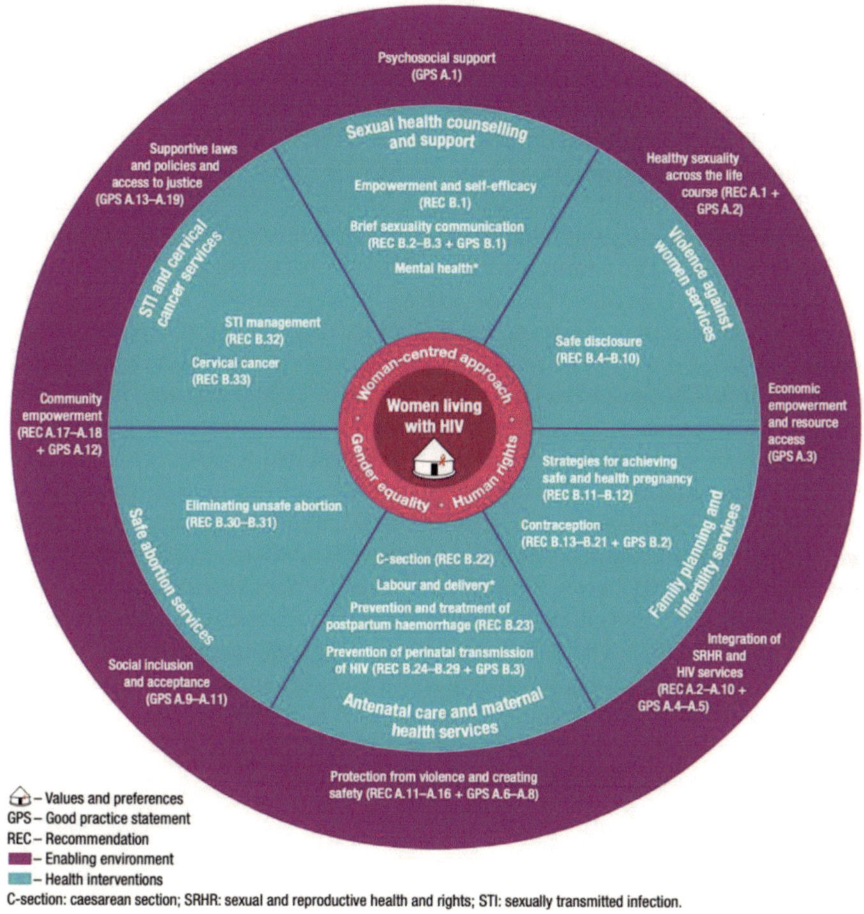


**Figure 1.**
*The framework of WHO recommendations and good practice statements to advance the sexual and reproductive health and rights of women living with HIV. Source: Consolidated guideline on sexual and reproductive health and rights of women living with HIV. World Health Organization; 2017.*

violence due to HIV diagnosis disclosure; social inclusion; promotion of community empowerment, and implementation of supportive laws and policies to access justice for violence victims and pregnancy termination decisions [56].

On a second front, for the specific health-related interventions relevant to the SRHR of WLHIV the guideline recommends the creation or improvement of health services (such as sexual health counseling and support for WLHIV), intended to provide self-efficacy and empowerment tools around sexual and reproductive health and rights; the prevention of sexually transmitted infections, and training of healthcare providers in sexual health based on rights knowledge. The guideline also suggests creating preventive services for violence against women supporting safe HIV diagnosis disclosure without stigma and discrimination [57]. Finally, regarding HIV-PT, the guideline recommends implementing friendly family planning services to provide comprehensive reproductive counseling. It advocates for planned and desired pregnancies avoiding unplanned pregnancies, with easy access to modern contraceptive methods based on the respect of sexual and reproductive options and rights of WLHIV, and safe abortion services for women who want a voluntary abortion. Within antenatal care and maternal health services, preventive strategies for HIV-PT, including antiretroviral treatments, delivery, and breastfeeding, are also emphasized [58, 59].

## 5. Conclusions

Women's differential vulnerabilities to HIV acquisition have been studied in different settings and are associated with disadvantageous economic security, education, and other structural determinants of health. HIV/AIDS affects especially young women who represent almost half of the new cases every year worldwide. Research has shown that WLHIV have significant unmet SRH needs, including differential SRH counseling, psychological support, protection from intrafamily and institutional violence, and family planning. HIV-PT is related to WLHIV's unmet SRH needs and access barriers. Lack of quality family planning counseling and low availability of modern contraceptive methods increase the risk of unplanned pregnancies and HIV-PT due to poor ART adherence and high attrition rates in prenatal care prenatal. WLHIV have better treatment adherence and a lower risk of HIV-PT and complications when pregnancies are planned and desired.

Additionally, SRH unmet needs in WLHIV are related to structural barriers and limitations to access good-quality services, imposing a limit to their capacity to make autonomous SRH decisions based on rights and leading to social exclusion, stigma, and discrimination. To improve the use and access to SRHS among WLHIV, the WHO released in 2017 a new guideline with evidence-based recommendations from a women-centered approach. The objective was to promote an enabling environment for WLHIV, with safe preventive interventions preserving healthy sexuality across the life course. It advocated for support for these women in making informed SRH decisions addressing restrictions and barriers from the inalienable right to women's health and wellbeing and as an essential part of the health strategies aimed for these populations.

## Author details

Marcela Gómez-Suárez
Research Division, Research Institute, Fundación Universitaria de Ciencias de la Salud (FUCS), Bogotá, Colombia

*Address all correspondence to: mgomez7@fucsalud.edu.co

## References

[1] Global Acceleration Action for the Health of Adolescents: guidance to support country implementation. Summary report. World Health Organization. 2017 (http://apps.who.int/iris/bitstream/handle/10665/255415/9789241512343-eng.pdf?sequence=1. accessed 4 January 2021).

[2] End inequalities. End AIDS. Global AIDS strategy 2021-2026. UNAIDS (https://www.unaids.org/sites/default/files/media_asset/global-AIDS-strategy-2021-2026_en.pdf accessed 7 March 2021).

[3] Barbosa R, Cabral C, do Lago T, Pinho A. Differences in the access to sterilization between women living and not living with HIV: results from the GENIH study, Brazil. PLoS ONE. 2016;11(11):1-18.

[4] Pinho A, Silva C, Barbosa R. Differences and similarities in women living and not living with HIV: contributions by the GENIH study to sexual and reproductive healthcare. Cad Saude Publica. 2017;33(12): e00057916.

[5] Kikuchi K, Wakasugi N, Poudel KC, Sakisaka K, Jimba M. High rate of unintended pregnancies after knowing HIV infection among HIV positive women antiretroviral treatment in Kigali, Rwanda. Biosci Trends. 2011;5(6):255– 63.

[6] Loutfy M, Raboud J, Wong J, Yudin M, Diong C, Blitz S, et al. High prevalence of unintended pregnancies in HIV-positive women of reproductive age in Ontario, Canada: a retrospective study. HIV Med. 2012;13(2):107-17.

[7] Buchanan AM, Cunningham CK. Advances and failures in preventing perinatal human immunodeficiency virus infection. Clin Microbiol Rev. 2009;22(3):493-507. doi:10.1128/CMR.00054-08.

[8] United Nations. Women's rights are human rights. Geneva: Office of the High Commissioner in Human Rights; 2014. Report No.: ISBN 978-92-1-154206-6.

[9] Consolidated guideline on sexual and reproductive health and rights of women living with HIV. World Health Organization. 2017 (https://www.aidsdatahub.org/sites/default/files/resource/consolidated-guideline-sexual-and-reproductive-health-and-rights-women-living-hiv-2017-full-report.pdf. accessed 4 January 2021).

[10] The Global HIV/AIDS Epidemic. KFF organization (https://www.kff.org/global-health-policy/fact-sheet/the-global-hivaids-epidemic/ accessed 7 January 2021).

[11] 20.1 million girls and women living with HIV. UNAIDS (https://www.unaids.org/en/resources/infographics/girls-and-women-living-with-HIV accessed 5 March 2021).

[12] Global HIV & AIDS statistics 2020 fact sheet. UNAIDS (https://www.unaids.org/en/resources/fact-sheet. accessed 4 January 2021).

[13] Women, girls, gender equality, and HIV. UNAIDS. Fact sheet. 2010 (https://www.ilo.org/wcmsp5/groups/public/---ed_protect/---protrav/---ilo_aids/documents/publication/wcms_152931.pdf. accessed 6 March 2021).

[14] Stirling M, Rees H, Kasedde S, Hankins C. Introduction: Addressing the vulnerability of young women and girls to stop the HIV epidemic in southern Africa. AIDS. 2008 Dec;22 Suppl 4: S1-3. doi: 10.1097/01.aids.0000341772.48382.57.

[15] Adimora AA, Ramirez C, Auerbach JD, Aral SO, Hodder S, Wingood G, El-Sadr W, Bukusi EA. HIV Prevention Trials Network Women at Risk Committee. Preventing HIV infection in women. J Acquir Immune Defic Syndr. 2013 Jul;63 Suppl 2(0 2): S168-73. doi: 10.1097/QAI.0b013e318298a166.

[16] Wira CR, Patel MV, Ghosh M, Mukura L, Fahey JV. Innate immunity in the human female reproductive tract: endocrine regulation of endogenous antimicrobial protection against HIV and other sexually transmitted infections. Am J Reprod Immunol. 2011 Mar;65(3):196-211. doi: 10.1111/j.1600-0897.2011.00970. x.

[17] Dunbar B, Patel M, Fahey J, Wira C. Endocrine control of mucosal immunity in the female reproductive tract: impact of environmental disruptors. Mol Cell Endocrinol. 2012;354(1-2):85-93. doi:10.1016/j.mce.2012.01.002.

[18] Wira CR, Fahey JV, Ghosh M, Patel MV, Hickey DK, Ochiel DO. Sex hormone regulation of innate immunity in the female reproductive tract: the role of epithelial cells in balancing reproductive potential with protection against sexually transmitted pathogens. Am J Reprod Immunol. 2010 Jun;63(6):544-65. doi: 10.1111/j.1600-0897.2010.00842. x.

[19] Roberts L, Liebenberg L, Barnabas S, Passmore JA. Vaginal microbicides to prevent HIV infection in women: perspectives on the female genital tract, sexual maturity and mucosal inflammation. Best Pract Res Clin Obstet Gynaecol. 2012 Aug;26(4):441-9. doi: 10.1016/j.bpobgyn.2012.02.002.

[20] Lai SK, Hida K, Shukair S, Wang YY, Figueiredo A, Cone R, Hope TJ, Hanes J. Human immunodeficiency virus type 1 is trapped by acidic but not by neutralized human cervicovaginal mucus. J Virol. 2009 Nov;83(21):11196-200. doi: 10.1128/JVI.01899-08.

[21] Thurman AR, Doncel GF. Innate immunity and inflammatory response to Trichomonas vaginalis and bacterial vaginosis: relationship to HIV acquisition. American journal of reproductive immunology. 2011;65(2):89-98.

[22] Powers KA, Poole C, Pettifor AE, Cohen MS. Rethinking the heterosexual infectivity of HIV-1: a systematic review and meta-analysis. Lancet Infect Dis. 2008;8(9):553-563. doi:10.1016/S1473-3099(08)70156-7.

[23] Heffron R, Donnell D, Rees H, et al. Use of hormonal contraceptives and risk of HIV-1 transmission: a prospective cohort study [published correction appears in Lancet Infect Dis. 2012 Feb;12(2):98]. Lancet Infect Dis. 2012;12(1):19-26. doi:10.1016/S1473-3099(11)70247-X.

[24] Adimora AA, Schoenbach VJ, Martinson FE, Coyne-Beasley T, Doherty I, Stancil TR, Fullilove RE. Heterosexually transmitted HIV infection among African Americans in North Carolina. J Acquir Immune Defic Syndr. 2006 Apr 15;41(5):616-23. doi: 10.1097/01.qai.0000191382.62070.a5.

[25] Gregson S, Nyamukapa CA, Garnett GP, Mason PR, Zhuwau T, Caraël M, Chandiwana SK, Anderson RM. Sexual mixing patterns and sex-differentials in teenage exposure to HIV infection in rural Zimbabwe. Lancet. 2002 Jun 1;359(9321):1896-903. doi: 10.1016/S0140-6736(02)08780-9. Erratum in: Lancet 2002 Oct 5;360(9339):1102.

[26] Wyatt GE, Myers HF, Williams JK. Does a history of trauma contribute to HIV risk for women of color? Implications for prevention and policy.

Am J Public Health. 2002;92(4):660-665. doi:10.2105/ajph.92.4.660.

[27] Zierler S, Feingold L, Laufer D, Velentgas P, Kantrowitz-Gordon I, Mayer K. Adult survivors of childhood sexual abuse and subsequent risk of HIV infection. Am J Public Health. 1991;81(5):572-575. doi:10.2105/ajph.81.5.572.

[28] Maman S, Campbell J, Sweat MD, Gielen AC. The intersections of HIV and violence: directions for future research and interventions. Soc Sci Med. 2000 Feb;50(4):459-78. doi: 10.1016/s0277-9536(99)00270-1.

[29] De Waal A, Klot J, Mahajan M.HIV/AIDS, security, and conflict: new realities, new responses. AIDS, Security, Conflict Initiative.2010. ISBN 978-0-9841257-9-1.

[30] Chandra-Mouli V, Armstrong A, Amin A, Ferguson J. A pressing need to respond to the needs and sexual and reproductive health problems of adolescent girls living with HIV in low- and middle-income countries. J Int AIDS Soc. 2015;18(Suppl 5):20297. doi:10.7448/IAS.18.6.20297.

[31] Gómez-Suárez M, Mello MB, Gonzalez MA, Ghidinelli M, Pérez F. Access to sexual and reproductive health services for women living with HIV in Latin America and the Caribbean: systematic review of the literature. J Int AIDS Soc. 2019;22(4): e25273. doi:10.1002/jia2.25273.

[32] Jewkes RK, Morrell R. Gender and Sexuality: Emerging Perspectives from the heterosexual epidemic in South Africa and implications for HIV risk and prevention. Journal of the International AIDS Society. 2010; 13:6.

[33] Abdool-Karim Q, Baxter C, Birx D. Prevention of HIV in Adolescent Girls and Young Women: Key to an AIDS-Free Generation. J Acquir Immune Defic Syndr. 2017 May 1;75 Suppl 1: S17-S26. doi: 10.1097/QAI.0000000000001316.

[34] De Bruyn M. Women and AIDS in developing countries. Soc Sci Med. 1992;34(3):249-62.

[35] Campbell C. Women, families & HIV/AIDS: a sociological perspective of the epidemic in America. Cambridge, UK: Cambridge University Press; 1999.

[36] Buzy JM, Gayle HD. The epidemiology of HIV & AIDS in women. In: Long D, Ankrah EM, editors. Women's experiences with HIV/AIDS: An International perspective. Columbia University Press Books; 1996. p. 181-204.

[37] Berer M, Ray M. Women, and HIV/AIDS, an international resource book. London: Pandora Press; 1993.

[38] Cullinane J. The domestication of AIDS: stigma, gender, and the body politic in Japan. Med Anthropol. 2007;26(3):255-92.

[39] Lawless S, Kippax S, Crawford J. Dirty, diseased & undeserving: the position of HIV positive women. Soc Sci Med. 1996;43(9):1371-7.

[40] Crossley M. Women living with long-term HIV diagnosis: problems, concerns, and ways of ascribing meanings. Women's Stud Int Forum. 1998;21:521-33.

[41] Chesney MA, Smith AW. Critical delays in HIV testing and care: the potential role of stigma. Am Behav Sci. 1999;42:1158-70.

[42] Green L, Ardon C, Catalan J. HIV, childbirth and suicidal behavior: a review. Hosp Med. 2000; 61:311-4.

[43] Heath J, Roadway MR. Psychological needs of women living with HIV. Soc Work Health Care. 1999; 29:43-57.

[44] Geter A, Sutton M, McCree D. Social and structural determinants of HIV treatment and care among women living with HIV infection: a systematic review: 2005-2016, AIDS Care: 2018;30:4, 409-416. doi:10.1080/09540121.2018.1426827.

[45] Cuca Y, Asher A, Okonsky J Kaihura, A, Dawson-Rose C, Webel A. HIV Stigma and Social Capital in Women Living With HIV, Journal of the Association of Nurses in AIDS Care: January 2017;28 (1): 45-54 doi: 10.1016/j.jana.2016.09.001.

[46] Paudel V, Baral KP. Women living with HIV/AIDS (WLHA), battling stigma, discrimination and denial and the role of support groups as a coping strategy: a review of literature. Reprod Health. 2015;12:53.doi:10.1186/s12978-015-0032-9.

[47] Gogna M, Pecheny M, Ibarlucia I, Manzelli H. The reproductive needs and rights of people living with HIV in Argentina: Health service users' and providers' perspectives. Social Science & Medicine. 2009.; 69(4): p. 813-20.

[48] Newman S, Grossman D, Blat C, Onono M, Steinfield R, Suzuki E. Does integrating family planning into HIV care and treatment impact intention to use contraception? Patient perspectives: HIV-infected individuals in Nyanza Province, Kenya. Int J Gynaecol Obstet. 2013; 13(Suppl): p. 6-23.

[49] Kim JC, Watts C. Gaining a foothold: tackling poverty gender inequality and HIV in Africa. Brit Med J. 2005;331:769-72.

[50] Gupta GR. Gender, sexuality, and HIV/AIDS: the what, the why, and the how. HIV/AIDS Policy Law Rev. 2000;5(4):86.

[51] Eliminating forced, coercive and otherwise involuntary sterilization: an interagency statement, OHCHR, UN Women, UNAIDS, UNDP, UNFPA, UNICEF and WHO. Geneva: World Health Organization; 2014 (http://apps.who.int/iris/bitstream/10665/112848/1/9789241507325_eng.pdf, accessed 6 March 2021).

[52] Gibbs A, Willan S, Misselhorn A, Mangoma A. Combined structural interventions for gender equality and livelihood security: a critical review of the evidence from southern and eastern Africa and the implications for young people. J Int AIDS Soc. 2012;15(3 Suppl 1):17362.

[53] Pronyk PM, Kim JC, Abramsky T, Phetla G, Hargreaves JR, Morison LA, Watts C, Busza J, Porter JD. Combined microfinance and training intervention can reduce HIV risk behavior in young female participants. AIDS. 2008;22:1659-66.

[54] Orza L, Welbourn A, Bewley S, Crone ET, Vazquez M; Salamander Trust. Building a safe house on firm ground: key findings from a global values and preferences survey regarding the sexual and reproductive health and human rights of women living with HIV. Geneva: World Health Organization; 2014 (http://salamandertrust.net/wpcontent/uploads/2016/09/BuildingASafeHouseOnFirmGroundFINALreport190115.pdf, accessed 6 March 2021).

[55] Bras M, Narasimhan M, Loutfy M, Khosla R (editors). Sexual and reproductive health and human rights of women living with HIV. J Int AIDS Soc. 2015;18(Suppl 5) (http://www.jiasociety.org/index.php/jias/article/view/20834/pdf, accessed 6 March 2021).

[56] Reproductive health strategy to accelerate progress towards the attainment of international development goals and targets. Global Strategy adopted by the 57th World Health Assembly. Geneva: World Health

Organization; 2004 (http://apps.who.int/iris/bitstream/10665/68754/1/WHO_RHR_04.8.pdf, accessed 6 March 2021).

[57] Integrating gender into HIV/AIDS programmes in the health sector: tool to improve responsiveness to women's needs. Geneva: World Health Organization; 2009 (http://www.who.int/gender/documents/gender_hiv_guidelines_en.pdf, accessed 4 January 2021).

[58] Preventing HIV and unintended pregnancies: strategic framework 2011-2015. The Inter-agency Task Team for Prevention and Treatment of HIV Infection in Pregnant Women, Mothers, and their Children; 2012 (http://www.who.int/reproductivehealth/publications/linkages/HIV_and_unintended_pregnancies_SF_2011_2015.pdf, accessed 6 March 2021).

[59] Global guidance on criteria and processes for validation: elimination of mother-to-child transmission of HIV and syphilis. Geneva: World Health Organization; 2014 (http://apps.who.int/iris/bitstream/10665/112858/1/9789241505888_eng.pdf, accessed 6 March 2021).

Section 2

# Advances in Treatment

Chapter 4

# Gender Differences in Human Immunodeficiency Virus (HIV) Disease Progression and Treatment Outcomes

*Fausta Mosha*


## Abstract

Several interventions have been implemented for control and prevention of HIV, including provision of Antiretroviral Therapy (ART). A major concern is how this investment can effectively reduce morbidity and mortality due to HIV given the existence of various factors that contribute to treatment failure. The purpose of this chapter is to elaborate the role of gender on HIV Disease progression and treatment outcomes. Demographic, epidemiological, clinical, immunological, treatment information as well as blood from HIV infected patients were collected. Epidemiological analyses, using standard phylogenetic and statistical tests were done. A follow-up of patients who were initiated on ART for 1 year enabled description of the gender differences in HIV disease progression and treatment outcome. After 1 year of follow up on ART, more females survived, and more females had undetectable viral load compared to males. However, women lost their initial immunological advantage as they presented with lower immunological recovery after 1 year of therapy. Socio-demographic factors do have an impact on disease progression during ART in HIV-1 infected patients. We recommend that more cohorts of patients be continuously followed up to understand the differences on ART outcome between males and females.


**Keywords:** gender differences, HIV, disease progression, treatment outcomes, Tanzania

## 1. Introduction

The epidemic of the Acquired Immune Deficiency Syndrome (AIDS) was first recognized as a clinical entity in 1981 [1]. HIV-1 was identified as the causative agent for AIDS in 1983 [2]. Globally, 37.9 million people were living with HIV, with 1.7 million new infections and 770,000 people having died of AIDS in 2018. Sub-Saharan Africa is the most severely affected by HIV infection in which 1 in every 20 adults (4.9%) are living with HIV [3].

HIV may be classified into types, groups and subtypes based on genetic similarities. There are two types of HIV: HIV-1 and HIV-2. Both types can be transmitted by sexual contact, blood contact, and vertical from mother to child [4]. HIV-1 is the predominant type worldwide with high genetic diversity due to extremely high mutation and recombination rates and high cell turnover [5]. The strains of HIV-1 can be classified into four groups: the "major" group M, the "outlier" group O and two new groups, N and P, representing the four separate introductions of simian immunodeficiency virus into humans [6]. The majority (more than 90%) of HIV-1 infections are caused by HIV-1 group M strains. Within group M there are nine genetically distinct subtypes (or clades) of HIV-1. These are subtypes A, B, C, D, F, G, H, J and K [7].

### 1.1 Gender differences in HIV disease progression

HIV disease progression and clinical manifestations of diseases may differ between women and men because of biological and socioeconomic factors [8]. The progression of AIDS reflects the chronic nature of the disease, the hallmark of which is a gradual deterioration of the host immune system. Previous investigations found different rates of HIV disease progression and of virological and immunological response to antiretroviral therapy (ART) among HIV-infected women compared with men [9]. The rate of increase in viral load over time is presumably greater for women than men given that women and men progress to AIDS and death at similar rates [10]. Baseline clinical and immunologic status was found to be predictors of HIV related mortality and morbidity in HIV outcome studies conducted in both high income and low-income countries. In the same studies, Men were found to have a significant higher rate of loss to follow-up and ART non-adherence [11]. More evidence suggests that HIV positive men have worse treatment outcomes than their women counterparts in Africa [12]. One study found that humans show strong sex differences in immunity to infection and autoimmunity, suggesting sex hormones modulate immune responses [13]. Similarly, evaluation of the gender difference in the outcome of other viral diseases like the COVID-19, revealed a higher mortality rate of male patients as compared with female patients, suggesting the protective role of estrogen [14].

Some studies have documented the differences in clinical progression of HIV between women and men due to hormones and age at the time of HIV infection [15], some studies suggesting that the differences in immunological responses to ART and mortality risk are due to biologic differences between men and women. The hormonal fluctuations in ovulating females, may affect immune function, and thus can cause variation on viral loads in women, where HIV RNA levels can decrease to a median of 0.16 log10 from the time of early follicular to the mid-luteal phase [10]. Studies involving male-to-female transsexuals have shown decrease in CCR5 expression when female hormones are administered.

Women living with HIV have limited access to care and treatment in several countries, most of who belong to ethnic or racial minorities, despite having better treatment outcomes and higher enrolment to ART care when compared to men [12]. However, women may delay ART initiation because of social obligations, pregnancy and socioeconomic factors [16].

### 1.2 Problem statement

Highly Active Antiretroviral Therapy (HAART) for treatment of HIV infection has improved the lives of HIV infected people by reducing the morbidity and mortality in patients receiving treatment. This has transformed a chronic fatal infectious disease into a manageable chronic infectious disease. Despite the use of HAART, numerous reports indicate failure of therapy due to lack of potency of some drugs or drug combinations, insufficient drug adherence and transmission of drug resistant virus. In a number of patients, HAART is not sufficiently effective thus results into virological, clinical and immunological decay [17]. The success of HAART in HIV infected patients may be influenced by other host factors; however, there is no enough information with combined assessment of a variety of factors that can influence treatment efficacy in clinical routine practice. One of the poorly understood factors that may influence disease progression and treatment response is gender. Men and women are affected differently with HIV and women's immune systems may respond differently to the virus because of hormonal influence. Women may also experience stronger side effects when using ARV drugs, such as central nervous system and gastrointestinal symptoms, which could then lower their ARV adherence [18]. Survival of HIV infected patient from the point of HIV diagnosis to AIDS within a comparable clinical care setting is affected mostly by the time of HIV diagnosis (WHO stage I and II), and other differences like age, gender, race and behavioral factors may also play a role on survival [19]. Also the differential use of ARV drugs for purely social economic reasons may lead to survival disadvantages for women [10].

Some patients, especially males diagnosed with HIV in developing countries, are not always successfully linked to onward treatment services, resulting in delays on initiating ART, or prophylaxis for opportunistic infections. Delayed presentation to care and treatment, and late HIV diagnosis, can result into late initiation of ART which affects adherence to treatment and results into poor prognosis in a disadvantageous group in the society [20]. More studies will be of benefit to explore the possibility of initiating ART at lower viral loads in women, especially during the early stages of infection.

### 1.3 Rationale of the study

As the use of ARV drugs in resource-limited countries increases, it is important to understand the effect of several factors on disease progression and outcome of ART. Combined analyses of various factors are scarce. Several studies except trials on specific regimens, have addressed aspects such as baseline clinical characteristics and adherence as predictors of treatment success. For limited resource settings, where ARV drugs are not sufficient for all patients, it would be cost effective to issue the drugs to patients who will ultimately adhere to the therapy. Cheap alternative methods are needed, to help in guiding therapy, especially in this era where the use of ARV has become widespread. If not controlled, emergence of HIV drug resistance will further complicate the epidemiology and transmission patterns of HIV especially during the time when ARV resources are limited. Various studies came up with different results on the survival difference between male and female HIV patients, and some of the differences were a result of inadequate medical care rather than biological differences. Some of the differences were related to the time to development of AIDS and opportunistic infections, viral load, ARV drug resistance and CD4 counts over time of observation. HIV disease progression can be determined by viral and host factors and sex differences in immune modulation. The purpose of this study was to assess the socio-demographic and virological factors predicting HIV disease progression among HIV patients in Dar es Salaam, Tanzania.

## 2. Methods

We conducted a cohort study in which we followed up HIV-infected ARV naïve patients for 1 year. We enrolled ARV naïve, HIV infected patients who were due to initiate ART, if they were 18 years and above, with available medical records from previous year. All patients were enrolled after providing written informed consent. We used a structured questionnaire to collect social demographic variables and anthropometric information, while patient record files and CTC database were used to collect data with respect to HIV diagnosis, clinical and ARV treatment information.

We categorized patients according to the clinical and performance scales of the staging system for HIV-1 patients [21]. The differences on these variables were assessed between males and females. All patients were followed up for a period of 1 year after starting treatment where treatment outcome was evaluated after 12 months from the time of initiation of therapy.

Ethical clearance to conduct the study was obtained from the National Institute for Medical Research in Tanzania and permission was seek from Hospital administration. All patient identifying information was de-linked from the collected data.

We collected blood in EDTA collection tubes, CD4 level was estimated using Becton Dickinson FACSCalibur, and viral load using TaqMan Viral-Load Assay COBAS® AmpliPrep.

Whole blood was separated by centrifugation at 4000 revolutions per minute for 20 minutes at −15°C, and plasma aliquoted and stored for testing. HIV RNA was extracted from plasma using Qiagen QIAamp Kit (Qiagen, Hilden, Germany) according to the manufacturer's instructions. cDNA synthesis was performed using SS III RT-PCR System (Life Technologies, USA) according to the manufacturer's instructions with the primers PrtM-F1 and RT-R1. Nested PCR was performed from obtained RT-PCR product, using primers Prt-F2 and RT-R2. The QIA quick PCR purification kit (Qiagen, Hilden, Germany) was used to purify the nested PCR products and quantified by agarose gel visualization. The ABI Prism Big Dye Terminator Cycle Sequencing Ready Reaction kit was used for sequencing together with the following primers PRT-F2, RT-R2, SeqF3 (35V), SeqR3 (90v1), SeqF4 (36V) and SeqR4 (AV44). Sequences were aligned using Clustal X [22], manually edited with BioEdit [23].

Data were analyzed using Epi Info version 3.5.1 and STATA 11. Clinical progression was assessed by comparing clinical characteristics at hospital registration, baseline and at the time of the study, taking into account the change in clinical characteristics over time. Median percentage weight gain was adjusted for amount of time on treatment. Gender differences were assessed using the Kruskal-Wallis test for continuous variables and the chi-square test for categorical data. Descriptive analysis was done for the basic demographic, clinical and immunological characteristics of patients as well as continuous variables like CD4 counts, age, plasma viral load levels and BMI for both males and females. Survival distributions for male and female patients were estimated using the Kaplan-Meier method. Patients who were lost to follow up were censored at the date when they were last seen. Patients who were still alive on the date when the study ended were censored on this date. Survival times were expressed in days. Cox's proportional hazards regression models were used to assess the associations between patient characteristics and outcomes. All other variables were included in multivariable models to assess their impact on the association between gender and outcomes.

## 3. Results

### 3.1 Sociodemographic characteristics

In a study of 234 patients recruited to initiate ARVs in Tanzania, 164 (70%) of them were females and 70 (30%) were males, with a refusal rate of 6 and 25%, respectively. Significantly more males had attended secondary schools than females; had a higher income and a better knowledge of ARV use (**Table 1**). There was no significant difference in median age (36 years), alcohol intake and use of traditional medicine and use of intravenous drugs (**Table 1**). Significantly more males tested for HIV following a chronic illness, in contrast to females who tested without signs of AIDS. Consequently, the disease stage at HIV diagnosis was significantly more advanced in males: more males had CD4 count <100 cells/ml at baseline; they had a significantly lower Body Mass Index and higher mean Log10 viral load (males 5.5; females 5.1) (**Table 1**).

### 3.2 Treatment response and disease progression

The prevalence of adherence to ART as measured by consistence in keeping appointment was not different between females (62.8%) and males (62.9%)

| **Characteristics** | **Females (N = 164)** | **Males (N = 70)** | **P value** |
|---|---|---|---|
| **Categorical variables** | **N (%)** | **N (%)** | |
| Primary level education | 156 (95.1) | 59 (84.3) | **0.005** |
| Above 100 US Dollar monthly income | 57 (34.8) | 43 (61.4) | **0.0002** |
| Having relative to remind to take medication | 133 (81.1) | 59 (843) | 095 |
| Alcohol intake | 33 (20.1) | 18 (25.7) | 04 |
| Use of traditional medicine | 97 (592) | 45 (652) | 05 |
| History of intravenous drug abuse | 8 (4.9) | 7(10) | 02 |
| Knowledge on ARV use and side effects | 10 (6.9) | 14 (20) | **0.005** |
| HIV testing due to chronic illness | 105 (64) | 55 (78.6) | **0.04** |
| Starting treatment with in 1 year of HIV diagnosis | 130 (793) | 55 (78.6) | 0.96 |
| Presence of 2 or more opportunistic infections | 75 (45.7) | 37 (519) | 03 |
| WHO staging at initiation of therapy | | | |
| Stage I | 16 (9.8) | 5 (7.1) | 0.6 |
| Stage II | 49 (29.9) | 16 (22.9) | 0.3 |
| Stage III | 82 (50.0) | 34 (48.6) | 0.8 |
| Stage IV | 17(10.4) | 15 (21.4) | **0.04** |
| CD4 < 100 cells/μl at ART initiation | 50 (333)* | 31 (47.0)* | **0.05** |
| **Continuous variables** | **Median (IQR)** | **Median (IQR)** | **P value** |
| Age (Years) | 35 (30.5–43.5) | 37 (33.5–42.0) | 0.38 |
| CD4 (cells/μl) at ART initiation | 149 (6–148; 75–218) | 102 (3–221; 47–184) | **0.02** |
| **Continuous variables** | **Mean (SD)** | **Mean (SD)** | **P value** |
| BMI at initiation of therapy | 22 (5) | 20 (4) | **0.002** |
| Log 10 viral load (RNA copies/ml) at initiation of therapy | 5.1 (1.3) | 5.5 (1.1) | **0.05** |

*Reproduced with permission from [24].*

**Table 1.**
*Baseline characteristics of 234 HIV-1 infected naïve patients, Dar es Salaam 2010.*

(**Table 2**). After 1 year of treatment with ART, the virological response was significantly better in females than in males (females 69%; males 45% with undetectable viral load) but the mean CD4 increase was significantly higher in males (230 cells/ml) than females (202 cells/ml) (**Table 3**).

The BMI was still significantly higher in females (24.5) compared to males (22.5), but the percentage increase of BMI was not significantly different. Also, more females (61.6%) survived than males (50%) with more deaths occurring in males. The unadjusted relative hazard for death for males at 1 year of ART was 1.94 with a confidence interval of 0.91 to 4.11, p = 0.08 (**Figure 1**). Cox proportional hazards (of a model containing social demographic variables) showed no significant difference in the survival rate after 1 year on treatment between males and females (relative hazard 1.02, 95% CI 0.75, 1.38). The reported opportunistic infections during 1 year of follow up were not significantly different (**Figure 2**).

### 3.3 Genotyping of patients with detectable viral load

A total of 67 patients were found to have detectable viral load at enrolment (females 43 (64%); Males 24 (36%)) during 1 year of treatment. Among which, 31 females and 29 males (60 total), were alive after 1 year of follow up. The status of 7 could not be confirmed after 1 year of treatment, as they were either died or Loss to follow up. The main subtypes identified were C 18 (27%), A 14 (21%) and D 13 (19%) (**Figure 3**). There was no significance difference on subtype distribution between males and Females.

#### *3.3.1 Nucleoside reverse transcriptase inhibitors (NRTI) resistance mutations*

A total of 6 (9%) patients had detected NRTI resistance mutations, 4 females and 2 males, among which 3 were alive after 1 year of therapy. There was no significance difference between males and females with regard to NRTI resistance mutations. Two of the patients had both NRTI and Protease Inhibitor (PI) resistance mutations. One patient-initiated treatment at WHO stage IV, four at WHO stage III and one at WHO stage II of disease staging. All patients started treatment with CD4 below 100 cells/μl and Viral Load above 5000 copies/ml.

#### *3.3.2 Non nucleoside reverse transcriptase inhibitors (NNRTI) resistance mutations*

A total of 2 (3%) patients had detected NNRTI resistance mutations, all females and were alive after 1 year of therapy. One patient-initiated treatment at WHO stage

| Characteristics | Females (N = 164) | Males (N = 70) | P value |
|---|---|---|---|
| | N (%) | N (%) | |
| Death | 21 (12.8) | 14 (20) | 0.2 |
| Alive | 101 (61.6) | 35 (50.0) | 0.1 |
| Lost to follow up | 42 (25.6) | 21 (30.0) | 0.5 |
| Missed appointments | 103 (62.8) | 44 (62.9) | 0.99 |

*Reproduced with permission from [24].*

**Table 2.**
*One year outcomes of 234 HIV infected patients after starting ART from September 2010 to August 2011.*

| Characteristics | Females (N = 101) | Males (N = 53) | P value |
|---|---|---|---|
| Percentage with undetectable viral load | 70 (69%) | 24 (45%) | **0.003** |
| **Continuous variables** | **Median (IQR)** | **Median (IQR)** | |
| CD4 (cells/µl) count after 1 year | 312 (252–413) | 321 (110–480) | 0.6 |
| **Continuous variables** | **Mean (SD)** | **Mean (SD)** | |
| Percentage BMI increase (from Baseline) | 10.5 (14.2) | 9.8 (17.5) | 0.3 |
| BMI after 1 year | 24.5 (4.8) | 22.5 (4.1) | **0.02** |
| Percentage weight gain | 10.4(14.3) | 9.3 (17.3) | 0.2 |
| CD4 (cells/µl) increase from baseline | 202 (516; 35–163) | 230 (272; 86–181) | **0.05** |

*Reproduced with permission from [24].*

**Table 3.**
*Progression of patients 1 year on ART, Dar es Salaam.*

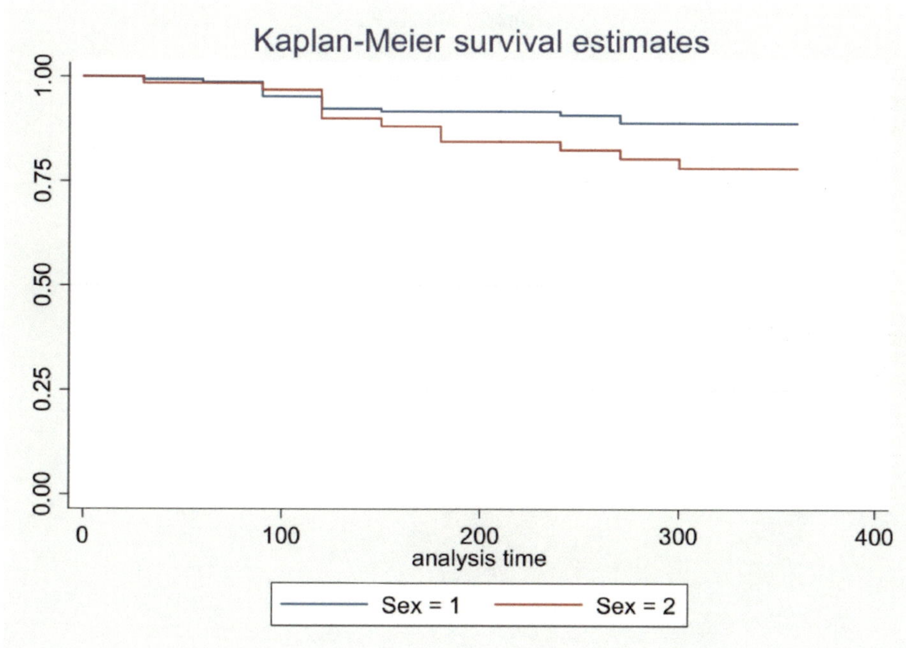


**Figure 1.**
*Kaplan-Meier survival curves on time to death for 234 patients, Dar es Salaam (reproduced with permission from [24]).*

III and one at WHO stage II of disease staging. All patients started treatment with CD4 below 100 cells/µl and Viral Load above 5000 copies/ml.

### *3.3.3 Protease inhibitors (PI) resistance mutations*

There was no patient with PI major resistance mutations. A total of 15 (22%) patients had detected PI minor resistance mutations, 6 females and 9 males, among which 6 were alive after 1 year of therapy. There was no significance difference between males and females with regard to PI minor resistance mutations. One patient-initiated treatment at WHO stage IV, nine at WHO stage III and five at WHO stage II of disease staging. Eight patients started treatment with CD4 below 100 cells/µl and all with Viral Load above 5000 copies/ml.

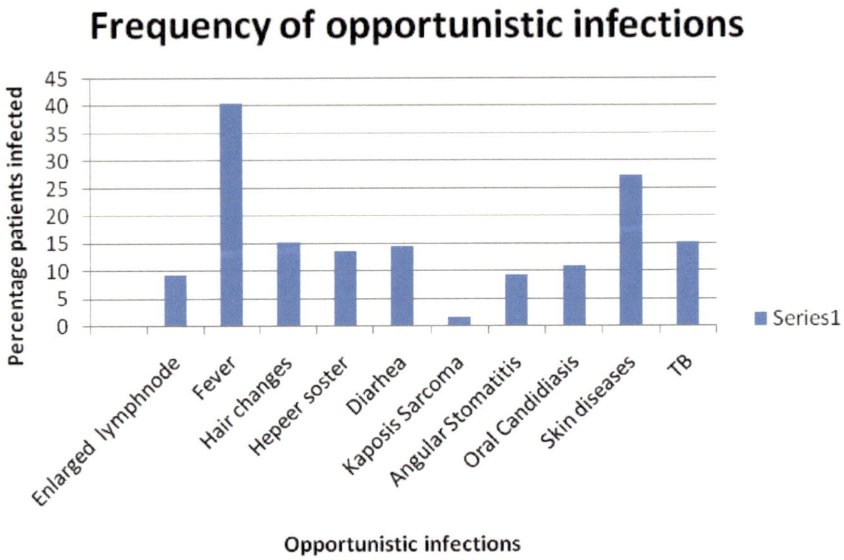


**Figure 2.**
*Observed opportunistic infection during 1 year of follow up (reproduced with permission from [24]).*

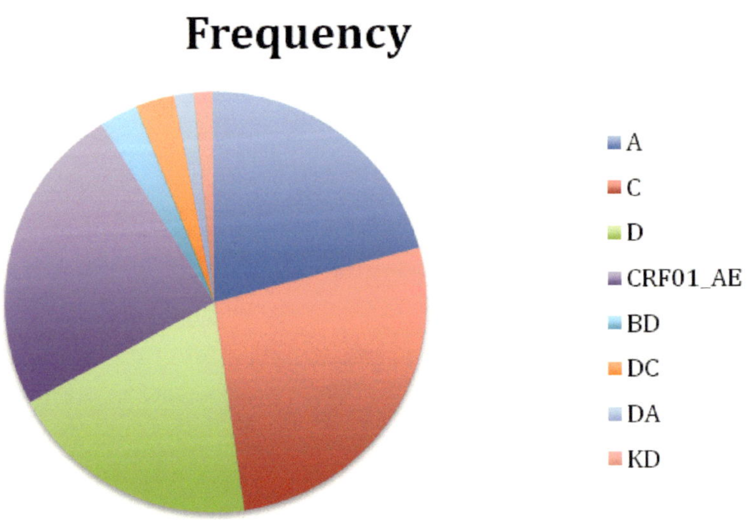


**Figure 3.**
*Subtype distribution of the detected sequences [24].*

## 4. Discussion

Our analysis of gender difference found significant clinical and social-demographic variations between females and males on HIV disease progression after 1 year of treatment. Overall, females were found to start CTC with higher CD4 count and BMI, and lower viral loads than males. Similar findings were reported by other studies, which found that women had higher CD4 cell count at ART initiation than men [9].

There was no statistical significant difference in survival between males and females in our study population after 1 year of follow up; this is in contrast with the findings of another study which found better survival among females and less disease progression among females after 3 years follow up [25]. The difference could be due to a shorter follow up (1 year) in our study compared to 3 years. Despite the fact that more males died, the ones who survived were found to have higher mean CD4 increase than females and more females had undetectable plasma viral load. Our findings are similar to a study, which found a significant better survival of female HIV-1 infected patients on HAART compared to male patients [10].

The fact that women did not fare worse than men is encouraging considering that females were found to be less educated with lower monthly income. This is consistent with the current data available in Tanzania where males earn more than females and are more educated [12]. However, males delayed reporting to care, with an advanced disease. Several studies have also indicated differences in health seeking behavior, between men and women, where more women were reporting to health facilities earlier [26]. This could be a result of differences in social responsibilities giving women more entry points to HIV services, like during pregnancy. However, we did not have similar results in this study.

The most common reason for HIV testing was presence of AIDS related symptoms, rather than voluntary testing, especially for males, and this denied the patients time for care at CTC. Despite the fact that both groups had delayed registering for care at CTC, 66% of males understood more about the use of ARVs than females. Immune Reconstitution Inflammatory Syndrome (IRIS) was associated with poor response to HIV patients initiated ART with low CD4 [26], which could also have happened to some of the patients in this cohort, as also observed in another study that CD4 cell count at ART initiation was a strong predictor of mortality [27].

Significant number of patients was using alternative medicines, illicit drugs and alcohol prior to starting ARVs, more observed among males than females. The use of alternative medicines and alcohol could contribute to the delay in seeking health care and late presentation to the care and treatment centers with advanced disease and also predispose the patients to poor adherence and poor prognosis [28]. However, there was no significant difference on ART adherence as measured by consistency in keeping appointment. There was also no significant difference in development of ARV drug resistance mutations. Excessive alcohol consumption can exacerbate immunosuppression, enhance the toxicity of ARV on liver cells and accelerating liver damage and may also depress the immune system leading to increased multiplication of the virus in mononuclear cells [29]. A significant number of patients reported use of injection-based illicit drugs in the past and present, this could have implications on ARV adherence and disease progression. Several studies have associated the use of illicit drugs with non-adherence to ART and poor prognosis. People who inject drugs (PWID) are also challenged with poor social and economic conditions, mental illnesses, which may affect their access and adherence to ART [30].

Women had a lower median viral load at initiation of therapy compared to men, despite the fact that there was no much difference on the period of illness before starting ART between the two groups. However, after 1 year of treatment, more females had undetectable plasma viral load and lower mean CD4 cell increase than males. This will need further evaluation, as this may need redefining the time to initiate ART in the two groups. Further studies are needed to understand the benefits of initiating ART, earlier with lower viral loads. This is because the absolute viral load seems to confer different risks for AIDS between men and women, which is not the case with relative viral loads [10]. Because HIV related morbidity is influenced by both viral and host factors, sex differences in immune modulation will likely play instrumental roles in determining the course of disease. Despite an observed high number of both males and females patients presenting with opportunistic infections; females reported more fever and oral candidiasis than males. The reason could be late presentation to CTC and thus could not benefit from the care and treatment services like prophylaxis against opportunistic infections. This may predispose the patients to poor prognosis and poor adherence after starting treatment [31]. Patients receiving HIV diagnosis late in the course of infection are usually more severely immune compromised and are more likely to present with co-morbidities like tuberculosis, which may be part of the immune reconstitution syndrome.

Consistent with our previous report, the most prevalent subtypes were A, C and D, and recombinants [32]. Our study found no contradiction to previous studies that found no association between subtype and therapy response, although our sample size was too small to conclude that [33].

Of concern was the detection of resistance to the first line ARV in Tanzania, in individuals who have been on treatment for only 1 year. This ARV resistance pattern was not limited to a particular subtype or gender. We observed minor PI mutations, which could be naturally occurring polymorphisms with no clinical significance. Interestingly, similar resistance mutations in the protease inhibitor genes were also observed in two different studies in Tanzania [34, 35].

## 5. Conclusion

We assessed the gender differences on HIV disease progression and outcomes after 1 year of ART among HIV infected patients and whether this potential difference is influenced by social, virological and immunological differences among patients starting ART. We observed some differences in clinical disease progression between males and females before starting ART and after 1 year of treatment. Male HIV patients delay seeking care and enter into treatment at a more advanced stage of HIV infection, which predisposed them to increased mortality. We also observed social factors that can affect future ART success in these patients. We recommend continuous follow up of this and other cohort of patients to understand responses to ART and the differences between males and females, together with advocating early HIV diagnosis and treatment to males. The observed gender difference between males and females will need further evaluation, as there may be a need to redefine the time to initiate ART in the two groups. The possibility of initiating ART at lower viral loads in women, especially during the early stages of infection merits further study. We recommend continuous follow up of this and more cohort of patients to understand responses to ART and the differences between males and females, together with advocating early HIV diagnosis and treatment to males.

It is important to monitor the viral response to patients on ART for early detection of treatment failure, together with understanding the ARV resistance pattern to ART Naïve patients and ART experienced patients. ARV resistance monitoring will help avoid unnecessary costs on use of ineffective treatment. The observed mutations within the pol region are of considerable concern because they may increase the development and spread of ARV resistant strains.

## Author details

Fausta Mosha
Ministry of Health Community Development, Gender Elderly and Children,
Dar es Salaam, Tanzania

*Address all correspondence to: fausta_mosha@yahoo.com

## References

[1] Gottlieb MS, Schroff R, Schanker HM, Weisman JD, Fan PT, Wolf RA, et al. Pneumocystis carinii pneumonia and mucosal candidiasis in previously healthy homosexual men: Evidence of a new acquired cellular immunodeficiency. The New England Journal of Medicine. 1981;**305**(24):1425-1431

[2] Barre-Sinoussi F, Chermann JC, Rey F, Nugeyre MT, Chamaret S, Gruest J, et al. Isolation of a T-lymphotropic retrovirus from a patient at risk for acquired immune deficiency syndrome (AIDS). Science. 1983;**220**(4599):868-871

[3] Statistics UG. UNAIDS GLOBAL Statistics. 2019 [cited May 2020]. Available from: www.UNAIDS.org

[4] Kanki PJ, Hopper JR, Essex M. The origins of HIV-1 and HTLV-4/HIV-2. Annals of the New York Academy of Sciences. 1987;**511**:370-375

[5] Overbaugh J, Bangham CR. Selection forces and constraints on retroviral sequence variation. Science. 2001;**292**(5519):1106-1109

[6] Plantier JC, Leoz M, Dickerson JE, De Oliveira F, Cordonnier F, Lemee V, et al. A new human immunodeficiency virus derived from gorillas. Nature Medicine. 2009;**15**(8):871-872

[7] Burke DS. Recombination in HIV: An important viral evolutionary strategy. Emerging Infectious Diseases. 1997;**3**(3):253-259

[8] Nicastri E, Angeletti C, Palmisano L, Sarmati L, Chiesi A, Geraci A, et al. Gender differences in clinical progression of HIV-1-infected individuals during long-term highly active antiretroviral therapy. AIDS. 2005;**19**(6):577-583

[9] Cornell M, Schomaker M, Garone DB, Giddy J, Hoffmann CJ, Lessells R, et al. Gender differences in survival among adult patients starting antiretroviral therapy in South Africa: A multicentre cohort study. PLoS Medicine. 2012;**9**(9):e1001304

[10] Gandhi M, Bacchetti P, Miotti P, Quinn TC, Veronese F, Greenblatt RM. Does patient sex affect human immunodeficiency virus levels? Clinical Infectious Diseases. 2002;**35**(3):313-322

[11] Hawkins C, Chalamilla G, Okuma J, Spiegelman D, Hertzmark E, Aris E, et al. Sex differences in antiretroviral treatment outcomes among HIV-infected adults in an urban Tanzanian setting. AIDS. 2011;**25**(9):1189-1197

[12] Druyts E, Dybul M, Kanters S, Nachega J, Birungi J, Ford N, et al. Male sex and the risk of mortality among individuals enrolled in antiretroviral therapy programs in Africa: A systematic review and meta-analysis. AIDS. 2013;**27**(3):417-425

[13] Kovats S. Estrogen receptors regulate innate immune cells and signaling pathways. Cellular Immunology. 2015;**294**(2):63-69

[14] Suba Z. Prevention and therapy of COVID-19 via exogenous estrogen treatment for both male and female patients. Journal of Pharmacy & Pharmaceutical Sciences. 2020;**23**(1):75-85

[15] Clark RA, Blakley SA, Rice J, Brandon W. Predictors of HIV disease progression in women. Journal of Acquired Immune Deficiency Syndromes and Human Retrovirology. 1995;**9**(1):43-50

[16] Mocroft A, Gill MJ, Davidson W, Phillips AN. Are there gender

differences in starting protease inhibitors, HAART, and disease progression despite equal access to care? Journal of Acquired Immune Deficiency Syndromes. 2000;**24**(5):475-482

[17] Oette M, Reuter S, Kaiser R, Lengauer T, Fatkenheuer G, Knechten H, et al. Epidemiology of transmitted drug resistance in chronically HIV-infected patients in Germany: The RESINA study 2001-2009. Intervirology. 2012;**55**(2):154-159

[18] Garcia de la Hera M, Ferreros I, del Amo J, Garcia de Olalla P, Perez Hoyos S, Muga R, et al. Gender differences in progression to AIDS and death from HIV seroconversion in a cohort of injecting drug users from 1986 to 2001. Journal of Epidemiology and Community Health. 2004;**58**(11):944-950

[19] Friedland GH, Saltzman B, Vileno J, Freeman K, Schrager LK, Klein RS. Survival differences in patients with AIDS. Journal of Acquired Immune Deficiency Syndromes. 1991;**4**(2):144-153

[20] Wolbers M, Bucher HC, Furrer H, Rickenbach M, Cavassini M, Weber R, et al. Delayed diagnosis of HIV infection and late initiation of antiretroviral therapy in the Swiss HIV cohort study. HIV Medicine. 2008;**9**(6):397-405

[21] WHO. Disease Staging System for HIV Infection and Disease. 2006 [cited 2016 25th August]. Available from: www.who.int

[22] Thompson JD, Gibson TJ, Plewniak F, Jeanmougin F, Higgins DG. The CLUSTAL_X windows interface: Flexible strategies for multiple sequence alignment aided by quality analysis tools. Nucleic Acids Research. 1997;**25**(24):4876-4882

[23] BioEdit [Internet]. 2009 [cited August 2016]. Available from: http://www.mbio.ncsu.edu/bioedit

[24] Mosha F, Muchunguzi V, Matee M, Sangeda RZ, Vercauteren J, Nsubuga P, et al. Gender differences in HIV disease progression and treatment outcomes among HIV patients one year after starting antiretroviral treatment (ART) in Dar es Salaam, Tanzania. BMC Public Health. 2013;**13**:38

[25] Morlat P, Parneix P, Douard D, Lacoste D, Dupon M, Chene G, et al. Women and HIV infection: A cohort study of 483 HIV-infected women in Bordeaux, France, 1985-1991. The Groupe d'Epidemiologie Clinique du SIDA en Aquitaine. AIDS. 1992;**6**(10):1187-1193

[26] Mugusi SF, Mwita JC, Francis JM, Aboud S, Bakari M, Aris EA, et al. Effect of improved access to antiretroviral therapy on clinical characteristics of patients enrolled in the HIV care and treatment clinic, at Muhimbili National Hospital (MNH), Dar es Salaam, Tanzania. BMC Public Health. 2010;**10**:291

[27] Alibhai A, Kipp W, Saunders LD, Senthilselvan A, Kaler A, Houston S, et al. Gender-related mortality for HIV-infected patients on highly active antiretroviral therapy (HAART) in rural Uganda. International Journal of Women's Health. 2010;**2**:45-52

[28] Kim TW, Kertesz SG, Horton NJ, Tibbetts N, Samet JH. Episodic homelessness and health care utilization in a prospective cohort of HIV-infected persons with alcohol problems. BMC Health Services Research. 2006;**6**:19

[29] Bagasra O, Bachman SE, Jew L, Tawadros R, Cater J, Boden G, et al. Increased human immunodeficiency virus type 1 replication in human peripheral blood mononuclear cells induced by ethanol: Potential immunopathogenic mechanisms. The Journal of Infectious Diseases. 1996;**173**(3):550-558

[30] Wood E, Montaner JS, Yip B, Tyndall MW, Schechter MT, O'Shaughnessy MV, et al. Adherence and plasma HIV RNA responses to highly active antiretroviral therapy among HIV-1 infected injection drug users. CMAJ. 2003;**169**(7):656-661

[31] Sabin CA, Smith CJ, Gumley H, Murphy G, Lampe FC, Phillips AN, et al. Late presenters in the era of highly active antiretroviral therapy: Uptake of and responses to antiretroviral therapy. AIDS. 2004;**18**(16):2145-2151

[32] Mosha F, Urassa W, Aboud S, Lyamuya E, Sandstrom E, Bredell H, et al. Prevalence of genotypic resistance to antiretroviral drugs in treatment-naive youths infected with diverse HIV type 1 subtypes and recombinant forms in Dar es Salaam, Tanzania. AIDS Research and Human Retroviruses. 2011;**27**(4):377-382

[33] Holguin A, Paxinos E, Hertogs K, Womac C, Soriano V. Impact of frequent natural polymorphisms at the protease gene on the in vitro susceptibility to protease inhibitors in HIV-1 non-B subtypes. Journal of Clinical Virology. 2004;**31**(3):215-220

[34] Nyombi BM, Holm-Hansen C, Kristiansen KI, Bjune G, Muller F. Prevalence of reverse transcriptase and protease mutations associated with antiretroviral drug resistance among drug-naive HIV-1 infected pregnant women in Kagera and Kilimanjaro regions, Tanzania. AIDS Research and Therapy. 2008;**5**:13

[35] Somi GR, Kibuka T, Diallo K, Tuhuma T, Bennett DE, Yang C, et al. Surveillance of transmitted HIV drug resistance among women attending antenatal clinics in Dar es Salaam, Tanzania. Antiviral Therapy. 2008;**13**(Suppl 2):77-82

Chapter 5

# Nanotechnology Based Drug Delivery for HIV-AIDS Treatment

*Inampudi Sailaja, Manoj Kumar Baghel and Ivvala Anand Shaker*

## Abstract

One of the biggest challenges of the world in this 21st century is to cure HIV-AIDS. In Present scenario different antiviral drugs are available in the market to reduce the worse condition and manage improved survival rate. These drugs are manageable but their bioavailability, lower permeability and poor half life of the drugs have limitations. If the drug is preferred in higher dosage in AIDS patients, the drug leads to toxicity and adverse effects to patients and increase resistant against HIV & if the drug is preferred in lower dose along with nano carriers it will reach the target area for beneficial effect, therefore drugs Lacking of Knowledge in Potent Drug delivery systems is due to instability, chemical degradation and tissue barrier difficulties are reasons to reach drug target successfully. In this scenario Nanotechnology based antiretroviral drugs delivery holds drug and will provide to cure AIDS. Nanotechnology based deliver system Nanocarriers like Liposomes, dendrimers, Nanoparticles, Polymeric Micelles, Nanovesicles, Nanoemulsion provide the way to deliver drug to targeting tissue. Nanobased carriers revolutionized the field of Pharmaceutics and Pharmaco Kinetic's in target drug delivery. The present study depicts nano based ARV drug provides increase efficiency with less adverse effects to control HIV. Like same way we can provide and increase nanobased drug delivery capacity to other available HIV drugs.

**Keywords:** HIV, AIDS, Antiretroviral Drugs, Nanocarriers, Nanotechnology, Drug delivery

## 1. Introduction

One of the most severe public health issues in the world is the Human Immunodeficiency Virus (HIV), the virus that causes Acquired Immunodeficiency Syndrome. HIV-AIDS remains one of the most difficult conditions to treat in the 21st century. However, multiple antiretroviral medications are present in the present situation, rendering the disease chronic rather than worse, which helps to improve the survival rate. According to the Statistical survey of WHO 2019 (World Health Organization), there are 38 million people living with HIV infection from that 1.7 million people newly added with HIV- infection in 2019 and 6.9 million people died from this 68% people accessed to Antiretroviral therapy [1]. In the late 20th century, it was reported that two strains of HIV diverge from SIV (Simian immunodeficiency Virus) from which HIV-1 spread across the world, and HIV-2 is more prominent in Africa [2]. HIV invades the mucosal membrane, destroys the immune system, leaving a wide variety of bacteria, viruses, fungi, protozoa vulnerable to infection in the host body. By exchanging body fluids due to blood transfusion, organ transplantation, physical intercourse, from affected parent to offspring, HIV infection propagates. One of the key sources of entry through the mucosal surfaces is the sexual transmission. The primary path of heterosexual HIV transmission is the female genital tract [3]. Sexual transmission via the rectal route is also a major issue that, due to its physiology, renders it more vulnerable to HIV infection [4]. Immune cells, i.e. macrophages and dendritic cells found in the sub-epithelial layer of the vagina or cervix mucosa are the main targets of HIV infection [5] in **Figure 1**.

During copulation, it moves by semen or other biological fluids that penetrate the stratified squamous epithelium or vaginal columnar epithelium to invade the target cell. HIV has a glycoprotein called gp120 on the surface of the viral coat, which attaches to the T-helper lymphocyte transmembrane protein receptor CD4 or chemokine receptor CCR5, CXCR4, and infects the cell [6]. Through endocytosis, HIV infects the host cell and fuses with the host cell membrane and releases into the host cytoplasm, it undergoes reverse transcription by incorporating proviral DNA into the host genomes. It then releases new viral particles that come out of it to infect the other cells. It infects macrophages and depletes the quantity of CD4+ cells that are the distinctive characteristics of an infection with HIV [7]. The use of multiple genes by HIV viruses (a) Main genes: gag, pol, and env (b) regulatory genes: tat, rev, nef, vif, vpr, and vpu, boost the productivity and hijacking the host's cellular system and develops its offspring to infect other cells [8]. Viral particles linger in the key after active infection in anatomical location such as dendritic cells,

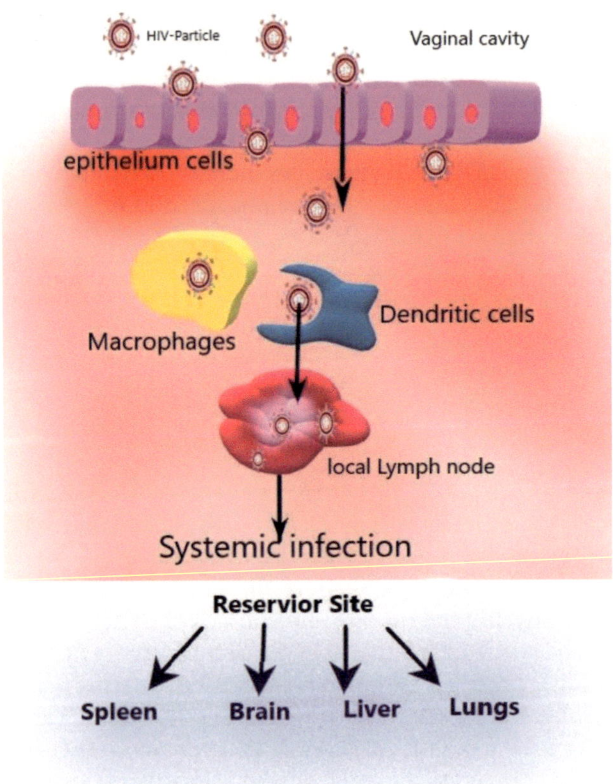


**Figure 1.**
*Pictorial representation of HIV particle invasion.*

macrophages, bone marrow, lymph nodes, spleen, lung, Central nervous system (astrocytes, microglial cells) [9–11]. When it remains in the CNS and induces a major loss in neural networks and eventually it leads to severe problems, such as HIV-associated dementia (HAD) If the patient is not, Well treated, it's going to die in 5–10 years (**Figure 2**) [12].

Various antiretroviral medications are used in the present scenario. Accessible in the market in a different mix, depends on the point of infection. High antiretroviral activity Therapy (HAART) is used to treat HIV/AIDS. It was introduced in 1996 and requires a mixture of at least three antiretroviral (ARV) medications. This treatment has been used to prolong the lifespan of HIV-infected patients [13]. However, this treatment is used to treat some of the infections Extension, but complete recovery has not yet been achieved as these ARV medications have certain drawbacks, such as mild water solubility, limited controlled release, low half-life reactivity, reduced blood barrier permeability, poor bioavailability is one of the major issues [14, 15]. ARV operates on the theory of blocking and inhibiting pathways, depending on the stage of the HIV cycle. Inhibitor of reverse transcriptase Blocks the action of the reverse transcriptase enzyme that prevents the conversion of viral RNA to DNA. Various nucleotide analogs drugs which incorporated in between the reverse Tran scripting chain in the host cytoplasm and terminate the process and non-nucleotide analogs drug bind to the reverse transcription enzyme and block the life cycle [16]. Various forms of AIDS treatment regimens are available that are available on the market. It has been prescribed. However, it is difficult to choose the right mixture of ARV products because of different considerations such as drug properties, drug tolerance status, patient reactivity, drug costing, drug toxicity, or some other adverse drug effect [17]. The biggest downside of the ARV treatment is the shorter period of availability in the bloodstream of the body in such a way that the viral particle at the location of reservoirs such as CNS, lymph nodes, and lungs

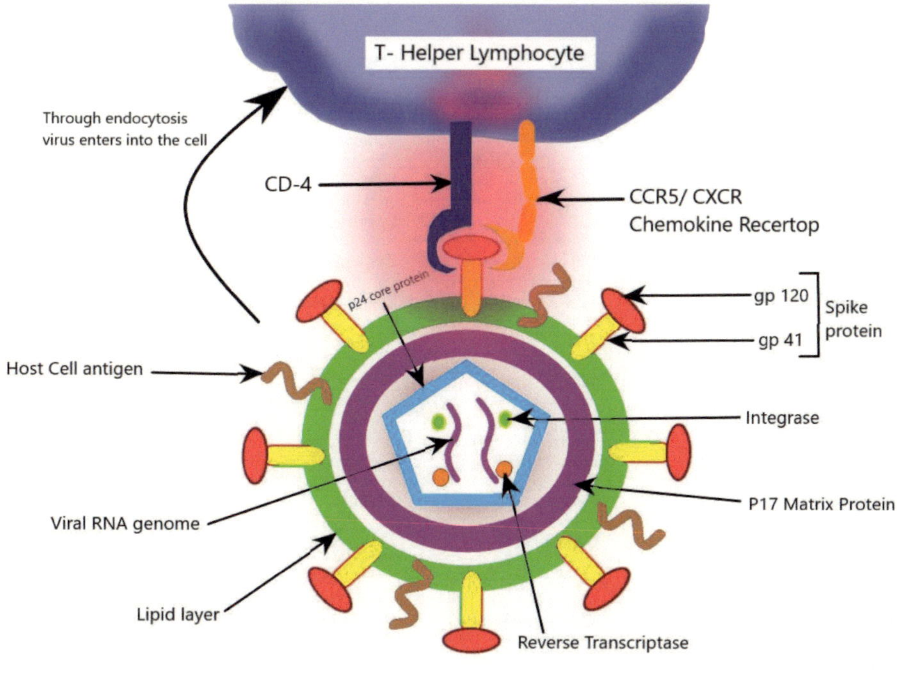


**Figure 2.**
*Pictorial art representing ligand receptor/co-receptor interaction between the HIV virus and Cd4 cell.*

is less exposed to the drug, such that higher doses of the viral particle are needed for a sustained period of time that develops resistance to the HIV strain [18]. The reservoir also includes latently infected cells, including CD4+ T-cells, Monocytes, macrophage lineage carrying incorporated transcription of the provirus silencing within the genome that might also re-infect the patient due to activation of the proviral genome [19]. In order to resolve such problems and drawbacks, nano-based drug delivery technologies, nano-medicines, and other nano-based strategies play a key role in drug effectiveness, drug reactivity, drug target accuracy, minimizing drug toxicity and negative impacts, and various major challenges currently facing ARV drugs in the present context.

## 2. Current anti-retro viral drug available in market for HIV-AIDS treatment

In present situation, HAART (Highly active anti-retroviral Therapy) regimen work on the principles by blocking replication process, reverse transcription, protein maturation process and viral-DNA integration process in to the host chromosomes. To inhibit this all process various class of drugs are available in the market which include Nucleotide reverse transcription inhibitors (NRTI), Non nucleotide reverse transcriptase inhibitors (NNTRI), integrase inhibitors, protease inhibitors as mention below in Error: Reference source not found (**Table 1**):

| **Non-nucleoside reverse transcriptase inhibitors (NNRTI)** | | | |
|---|---|---|---|
| **Generic names** | **Abbreviations** | **Brand name** | **Manufacturer** |
| Efavirenz | EFV | Sustiva® | Bristol-Myers Squibb |
| Etravirine | TMC125 | Intelence® | Tibotec |
| Nevirapine | NVP | Viramune® | Boehringer Ingelheim |
| Delavirdine | DLV | Rescriptor® | ViiV Health care. |
| **Reverse transcriptase inhibitors (NRTI)** | | | |
| Didanosine | ddI | Videx® | Bristol-Myers Squibb |
| Zalcitabine | ddC | HIVID® | Roche |
| Lamivudine | 3TC | Epivir® | GlaxoSmithKline |
| Abacavir | ABC | Ziagen® | GlaxoSmithKline |
| Zidovudine | AZT | Retrovir ® | GlaxoSmithKline |
| Tenofovir | TDF | Vemlidy® | Gilead Sciences |
| Stavudine | d4T | Zerit® | Bristol-Myers Squibb |
| **Integrase inhibitors** | | | |
| **Generic names** | **Brand name** | **Manufacturer** | |
| Raltegravir | Isentress® | Merck | |
| Dolutegravir | Tivicay® | ViiV Health care. | |
| **Protease inhibitors** | | | |
| **Generic names** | **Abbreviations** | **Brand name** | **Manufacturer** |
| Saquinavir | SQV | Invirase® | Roche |
| Atazanavir | ATV | Reyataz® | Bristol-Myers Squibb |
| Indinavir | IDV | Crixivan® | Merck |

| | | | |
|---|---|---|---|
| Nelfinavir | NFV | Viracept® | Agouron Pharmaceuticals |
| **Drug combination** | **Brand name** | **Manufacturer** | |
| Lopinavir + Ritonavir | Kaletra® | Abbott Labs | |
| Lamivudine + Zidovudine | Combivir® | GlaxoSmithKline | |
| Abacavir + Lamivudine | Trizivir® | GlaxoSmithKline | |
| Tenofovir + Emtricitabine | Truvada® | Gilead Sciences | |
| lamivudine + tenofovir disoproxil fumarate | Temixys® | Celltrion | |

**Table 1.**
*Market Available ARV drugs for HAART.*

## 3. World of Nanobiotechnology in field of drug delivery

The field of Nanobiotechnology that emerges with the great modern manufacturing for higher performance of drug due the scope of the Nanoscale process (1-100 nm). With the advent of nanotechnologies, it revolutionizes drug delivery in the field of pharmaceuticals. The fundamental theory is to modulate the pharmacokinetics of the chemical molecule that has deserved to eliminate HIV from the body without damaging the body. It also increases the bio-distribution and bioavailability of the drug to expose the virus particle for a longer duration with a higher goal precision. Being Nano-sized, the Nano-material drug reacts differently than the conventional drugs, because of their decrease in scale and, they have a healing impact within the living environment.

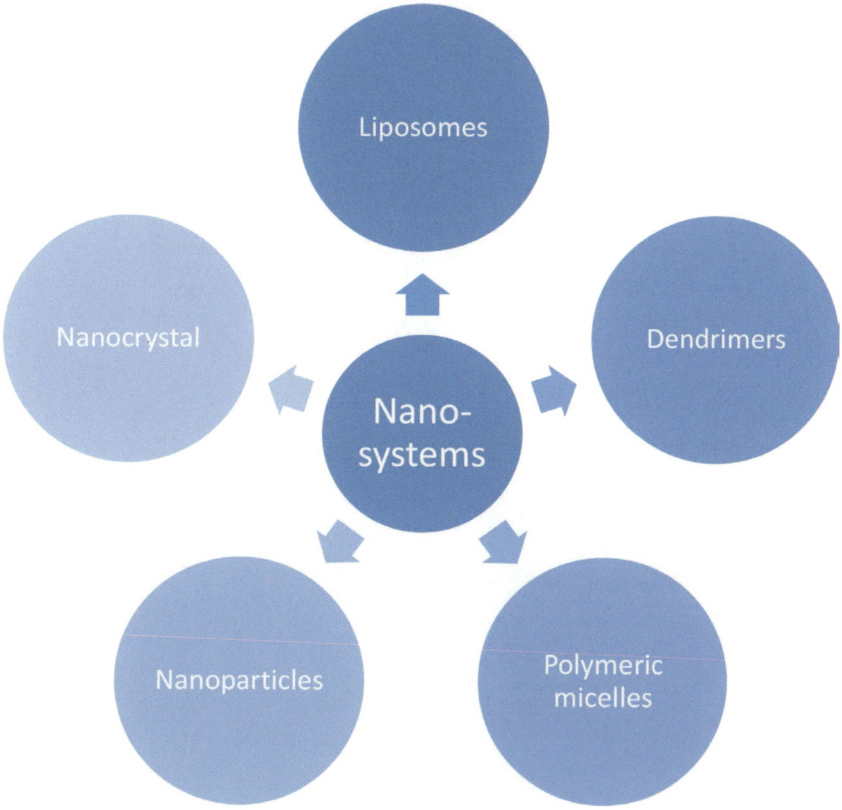


**Figure 3.**
*Pictorial representation of Different Nano-systems.*

The encased drug carried by the Nano-systems governs its, absorption, distribution, and excretion on the basis of its surface charges present on the Nano-systems due to its physical and chemical properties [20, 21]. Application of nanotechnology to the delivery of ARV drugs Holds the potential to treat AIDS and it could be beneficial Drugs at the anatomical reservoir site and also raise the half-life of drugs [22]. It has become possible to use nanotechnology for increased delivery of badly water-soluble drugs, selective delivery of drugs to particular cells or tissues, Intracellular transmission of macromolecules [23]. Nano-carriers give a range of advantages, such as control of drugs degradation, drug specificity and delivery of biological products molecules, such as proteins, peptides, oligopeptides, oligonucleotides, etc. Nanocarriers are now using it to solve the limitation of therapeutic uses, such as drug delivery, bioavailability of drugs, drug conformation stability, physicochemical stability, improved transmission permeability, drug clearance, cellular absorption, reduction of immunogenic reaction (**Figure 3**) [24, 25].

Different Nano-system strategies can be utilized as shown in the Error: Reference source not found for ARV drug entrapment which holds to cure HIV infection.

## 4. Liposomes

Liposomes became the first type of Nanomaterial in 1976, functionalized for drug delivery applications [26]. A liposome is a tiny microscopic vesicle that is made up of the phospholipid bilayers that are normally encircled by the watery centre. It is beneficial to hold hydrophilic drugs by trapping with in the centre, while the hydrophobic drug is inserted into the lipid bilayer [27]. The scale of the liposomes can be between 25 nm and multiple microns, offering the benefit of permeability (**Figure 4**).

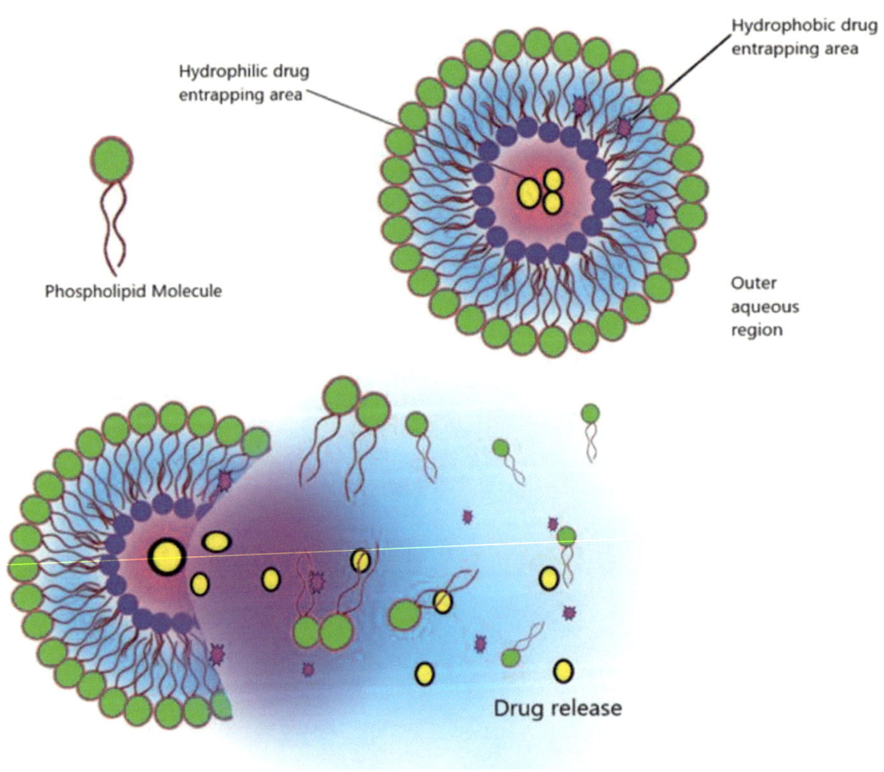


**Figure 4.**
*Pictorial art of Liposomes for targeted drug delivery.*

Human or synthetic phospholipids, along with cholesterol and additionally lipids, protein or peptide fragments, are used in their preparation. Liposomes, upon entering the living organism, realize that they are alien particles surrounded by mononuclear phagocytic cells, such as macrophages, so that liposomes are a beneficial carrier of the anti-HIV drug to the infected cell. As a result, liposomes can increase the effectiveness of the anti-HIV medication by lowering its side effect [28]. There are three types of liposomes, namely small uni-lamellar vesicles, large uni-lamellar vesicles, and multi-lamellar vesicles. In their natural form, liposomes are trapped by the reticulo-endothelial system and easily clear from circulation. Liposomes interact with the cell surface in a number of ways. The first is lipid exchange, which helps to exchange lipid molecules between liposomes and cell membranes. The second is adsorption, which diffuses across the cell membrane in the encapsulated substance within the liposome. Third, liposomes can, by fusion, transfer their encapsulated material to the cell membrane [29]. And foremost important characteristic of liposomes, it is engulfed up by the cell through endocytosis [30].

### 4.1 Liposomal ARV drug formulation for anti-HIV effect

Zidovudine drug is reverse transcriptase inhibitor which is amphiphilic drug, loaded into liposomes resulted in major improvements in the pharmacokinetic properties and distribution of tissues, including higher levels of distribution in reticulo-endothelial system and brain organs, longer half-life and lower average clearance of it relative to conventional zidovudine solution. Therefore, the approach to pro-drug liposomes can lead to reduced toxicity and improved efficacy of zidovudine-based HIV therapy [28]. The liposomal loaded zalcitabine system (2′,3′-dideoxycytidine, ddc) was examined in a mouse macrophage cell line that demonstrates high intracellular absorption due to anionic loading of liposomes [31]. The liposome of the phosphorylated form of zalcitabine, tested it in a murine-acquired immunodeficiency syndrome model that arrays chemical stability, improved retention entrapment, and decreased viral load in the mononuclear phagocyte system in both spleen and bone marrow [32]. Several in vitro and in vivo experiments have been undertaken by trapping ARV drugs such as acyclovir, indinavir, zidovudine, and lamivudine into the permuted liposomal structure, which shows 12 folds higher amount in blood plasma as compare to conventional drug by utilizing elastic liposomes in rat model, skin permeation of zidovudine improved 18-fold relative to simple drugs, this indicates a high effectiveness of transdermal flux relative to free drugs and higher deposition in the reticulo-endothelial organ system following the launch of zidovudine-loaded elastic liposomes trans-dermal. This suggests a greater permeability of the liposomal composition in rat model [33]. For lymphatic's targeting, the surface of liposomes was coordinated by charges and site-specific ligands to facilitate lymphatic, prominently lymph node and spleen localization. The particle-charged liposomes were formed using stearylamine, dicetyphosphate, and mannose conjugate. Evaluating these three compounds, fluorescent microscopy indicates a greater position of mannose conjugate than negative or positive liposomes, this shows the enhanced targeting of lymphatic's in AIDS chemotherapy [34]. Liposomes are quickly phagocytised by macrophages, in order to improve the extended circulation time and bioavailability of the drug the surface is changed by hydrophilic molecules such as polyethene glycol, PEGylated liposomes with targeting ligand derived from HIV gp120 guided monoclonal antibody F10 and seen as novel approaches to the battle against HIV-1. These Nano-immuno-liposomes display greater and longer antiviral efficacy than free drugs or drugs that encapsulate non-targeted liposomes [35]. Magnetic liposomes containing azidothymidine 5′-triphosphate, the average size of these magnetic liposomes 150 nm, are prepared using phosphatidylcholine and cholesterol with a magnetite loading efficiency of 54 per cent and 45.3 per cent. It is researched to verify transmigration through the in vitro blood–brain barrier model and monocyte mediated transport by adding external magnetic field. The outcome of the apparent permeability of magnetic azidothymidine liposomes was 3 times higher than free azidothymidine [36]. Indinavir filled with mannosylated liposomes containing βD-1 Thiomannopyranoside residues covalently coupled to dimyristoyl Phosphatidyl ethanolamine (DMPE), which was also incorporated with di-steroylphosphatidyl-choline and cholesterol, was used to attack the mononuclear phagocyte function (J774.A1 macrophage cell line). This liposome showed approximately 88.7 per cent of entrapment efficacy. Important levels of the drug have been identified in macrophage rich tissues such as the liver, spleen, and lungs relative to liposomes and free drugs [37]. Cell-derived liposomes demonstrate greater and more effective targeting. It is orchestrated from the cytoplasmic membranes of the cell expressing CCR5, the human receptor for gp120 located mainly on the surface of HIV-infected cells and HIV-virion, which display a substantial 60% reduction in the viability of the HIV-infected model cell due to binding and nullifying infectivity [38]. PEGylated liposomal transmission to mammalian cells in culture demonstrated sustained release with encapsulation efficiency of approximately 33 per cent. In cell viability tests of Jurkat T- cell, lower cytotoxicity was found relative to non-PEGylated liposomes [39]. Immune-liposomes filled with heparin active serine Antithrombin III (hep-AIII) protease inhibitor injected into the non-human primate system model. The outcome indicates a steady decrease of more than 1(10) log in plasma viral load that concludes hep-AIII as a rescue or replacement agent for HIV strain immune to standard ARV drugs [40]. Glycan-Modified HIV NFL Envelope Trimer-Liposome vaccine formulation showed broad generation of neutralizing Antibody in modal, which hold proof for immunogenic vaccine development to combat AIDS [41]. The use of liposomes to prevent the spread of HIV through sexual transmission has been confirmed. The structure of the mixture consisted of liposomes that acted as decoys allowing the HIV virus to bind to liposomes instead of host cells. Some formulations contain un-conjugated liposomes whose physicochemical properties make it possible to bind to the HIV virus or to change the ligand that binds to the HIV virus has also been documented. The liposomes were created from lipids picked from the community consisting of cationic lipids, anionic lipids, neutral lipids, zwitter ionic lipids, and various combinations.

### 4.2 Dendrimer

The dendrimer consists of Dendron's, a small branching unit that includes an internal and a periphery end group, a polymeric nanostructure consisting of multiple branching units in a layer by layer pattern that characterizes the size, growth and microenvironment within it (**Figure 5**) [42].

Dendrimer contains space within the Dendron that can be used for drug trapping, selective drug release, defense against environmental destruction, precise targeting. Dendrimer with significant numbers of peripheral groups and inner cavities are possible vectors for chemical drugs, peptides and HIV inhibition genes. These compounds are either capable of interacting with peripheral groups or are encased in dendrimer cavities with hydrogen bonds, electrostatic and hydrophobic interactions [43, 44]. Dendrimers can improve the stability of chemical drugs and encourage cellular absorption by functional end-groups. In the case of gene therapy, Dendrimers can take the place of viruses to transfer interference genes to target cells to suppress replication of HIV. The scale of the dendrimer is less than 100 nm with less poly dispersity and higher functionality than the traditional polymer with the 3-Dimensional architecture. The kernel can be synthesized by ammonia and

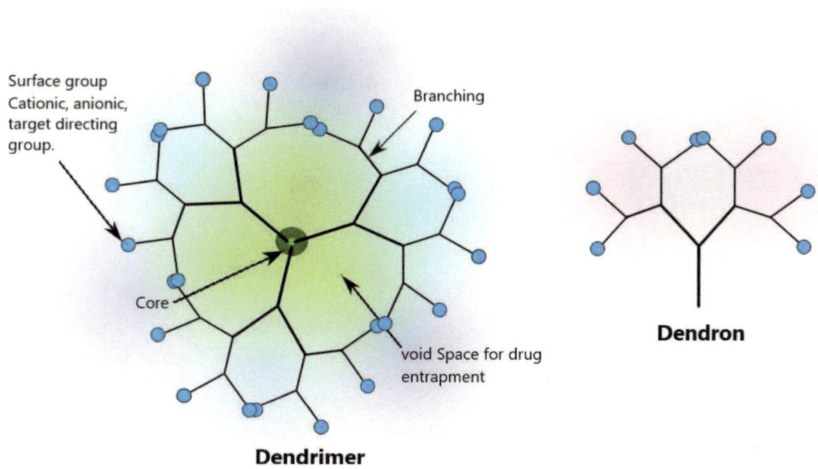


**Figure 5.**
*Pictorial art of dendrimer complex for drug delivery.*

ethylene diamine encircling highly branched repeaters such as polyether, porphyrins, poly-amido-amines, polyphenyl and polyamine acids. Core shell properties are mainly based on multivalent surfaces that contain targeting or functional groups. Dendrimers have been engineered to interact with unique functional end-groups preferably with HIV envelope proteins and receptors on host cells in order to inhibit the combination of HIV and host cells and later stages of HIV replication.

### 4.3 Dendrimer formulation for targeting HIV-AIDS

Following the discovery of the HIV inhibition process, two poly anionic Dendrimers BRI2932 (SPL2923) and BRI6195 (SPL6195) were found to inhibit the replication of HIV (strain IIIB) in the EC50 at 0.1 and 0.3 μg/mL, respectively, with exceptionally low cytotoxicity in the host cells. The gp120 binding assay and the virus adsorption assay showed that both substances had an effect on the docking of HIV in the host cells. In addition, higher concentrations of SPL2923 (500–2500 times EC50) could also block later stages of HIV infection. Correspondingly, the findings of cellular uptake studies revealed that SPL2923 was capable of intrusion into the host cell, while SPL6195 was not [45].

Anti-HIV medication Efavirenz loaded with tuftsin-conjugated fifth-generation poly (propylene imine) (T5PP) dendrimer, which reveals the prolonged action of the treatment in 24 hours, negligible cytotoxicity and cellular absorption 34.5-fold stronger than the free in vitro drug in infected macrophages [46]. Dendriplexes produced by 2G-NN16 and siRNAs were used for brain targeting. Transfection efficiency assessment and transcytosis by means of an in vitro blood–brain barrier (BBB) model on astrocytoma cells (U87MG). Unexpectedly, Dendriplexes developed at a ratio of 2G-NN16/siRNA of 8 displayed the highest transfection efficiency. The siRNAs-dendriplexes have been shown to effectively cross the monolayer barrier. Dendriplexes demonstrated a dose-dependent HIV inhibition of up to 85 per cent of HIV infected U87MG cells [47].

Water-stable cationic carbosilane dendrimers, which are used for drug distribution in the HepG2 cell line and PBMC, display greater interaction with nucleic acid through the development of nanoconjugates in different stable pH ranges. Nanoconjugates also display a high degree of transfection with oligonucleotide anti-HIV in laboratory settings [48]. SPL7013 is one of the anionic dendrimers that

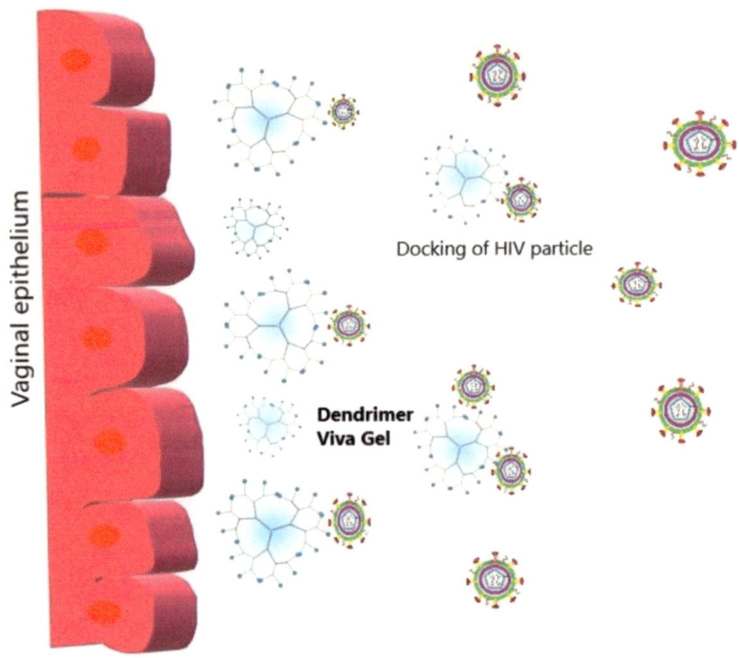


**Figure 6.**
*Pictorial representation of working function of Viva gel, a tropical microbicide.*

contains the divalent benzhydryl amide of L-lysine as the nucleus of naphthalene sulfonic acid. Efficacy tests of 5% w/w SPL7013 as an aqueous gel found that the single intravaginal dose of the formulation shielded pigtailed macaques from infection with the intravaginal (SIV) simian-human immunodeficiency virus [49]. Multivalent phosphorous-containing catanionic dendrimers with galactosyl ceramide analogs have a significant affinity to the V3 loop of the HIV-1 viral envelope protein gp120, which inhibits viral fusion with the plasma membrane and thus serves as an entry inhibitor [50]. Dendrimer may also be considered a potent factor in the selective expulsion of HIV.

### 4.4 FDA approved dendrimer of AIDS

A tropical microbicides, first dendrimer-based drug called VivaGel® has been submitted to the US FDA as an investigational novel drug, an aqueous-based polyacrylic acid gel containing SPL7013 buffered to physiological pH, a nanoscale dendrimeric molecule that binds to viruses and stops them from affecting the body's cells [51] as mention in **Figure 6**.

## 5. Nanoparticles

Nanoparticles are small colloidal particles of size ranges (10-100 nm) [52]. They have the ability for precise targeting of drugs with controlled release, depending on their size and polymer structure. Nanoparticles are expected to improve the composition and effectiveness of medications with some physiochemical weakness of low stability and solubility [53]. Owing to their scale, nanoparticle-based therapies can conveniently be performed using a range of methods (i.e., intravenous, subcutaneous, intraperitoneal) and can pass body barriers [54]. Nanoparticles have increasingly experimented with selective delivery of ARV drugs to achieve modulated pharmacokinetics, improved potency, reduced systemic toxicity, and adverse effects.

### 5.1 Polymeric nanoparticles

A polymeric nanoparticle can be produced as per a favorable approach to the targeted delivery of ARV drugs. Various polymers are used for the construction of anti-HIV polymeric nanoparticles such as poly (lactic acid) (PLA), poly (lactic-co-glycolic acid) (PLGA), poly (alkyl) cyanoacrylate, poly (ethylene glycol-co-(lactic-glycolic acid)), poly(caprolactone), and poly(methyl) methacrylate. PLA and PLGA have been evaluated and considered safe for human use by the FDA. Various drugs can be integrated into these polymers on the basis of their hydrophilicity or hydrophobicity, and release properties can easily be changed on the basis of specifications.

Zidovudine-loaded polyvinylpyrrolidone (PVP)/stearic acid (SA)-polyethylene glycol (PEG) nanoparticles (PSNPs) have been formed using a solvent-emulsifying evaporation process. And tested in vitro murine neuro-2a and HeLa cells, which display substantial change in cell internalization, stable colloidal suspension, enhanced cell absorption, increased half-life, with no cytotoxicity [55]. Saquinavir-loaded poly (ethylene oxide)-modified poly (epsilon-caprolactone) (PEO-PCL) nanoparticle method using a solvent displacement technique. Cellular absorption and bio-distribution of PEO-PCL are studied in vitro in human monocyte/macrophage (Mo/Mac) THP-1 cell line, which results in a higher accumulation of drugs than in aqueous phase form [56].

Electromagnetic intrusion in the permeability of Saquinavir charged nanoparticles studied in human brain micro vascular endothelial cells. Here Nanoparticles are used as polybutylcyanoacrylate (PBCA), metylmethacrylate-sulfopropyl-methacrylate (MMA-SPM) for the study of a human blood–brain barrier model that offers higher permeability coefficient across the blood–brain barrier [57]. The Chitosan-based nanoparticles loaded with tenofovir were developed to optimize its muco adhesion. By decreasing the size from 900 nm to 188 nm of nanoparticle, non-cytotoxicity to the vaginal epithelial cell line with improved muco adhesion 6 percent to 12 percent was reported [58]. This represents polymeric nanoparticles demonstrate successful drug delivery in the fight against HIV (**Figure 7**).

### 5.2 Solid lipid nanoparticles (SLN) and nano-structured lipid carriers (NCL)

SLN is a thin microscopic structure consisting of physiological lipids that form stable Nanoparticles of aqueous surfactant solution. SLN provides a great opportunity to mount ARV drugs because of its small scale, high drug loading ability, slow degradation of lipid matrices, large surface reactivity. SLN also promotes sustained release, minimizing drug toxicity, dosing frequency and fluctuation of plasma drug levels. SLN shows biphasic drug release due to its composition, initial burst due to its surface adsorption, and steady release from its lipid center due to progressive degradation [59, 60]. SLN of atazanavir-name protease inhibitors was developed by Chattopadhyay et al. to verify permeability and, a blood–brain barrier model was tested on the human brain micro vascular cell line (hCMEC/D3) that successfully results from a higher accumulation of the drug by endothelial cell monolayer than the aqueous drug solution with obvious permeability across the barrier membrane [61]. Zidovudine palmitate loaded SLN, which accommodates tri laurin as a lipid center with a combination of dimyristoyl phosphatidylglycerol resulting in neutral charging. It is then modified with polyethene glycol moieties and higher surface

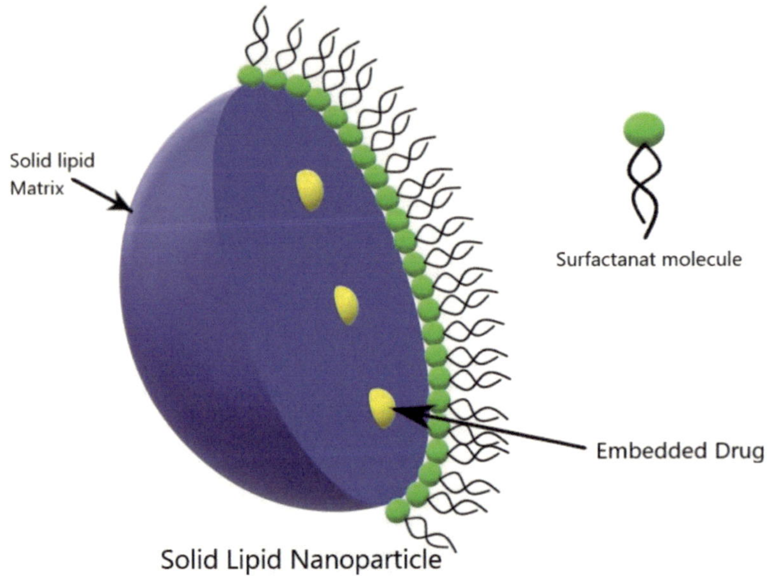


**Figure 7.**
*Pictorial art of Solid lipid Nanoparticle carrying embedded drug.*

phospholipids resulting in better plasma circulation with increased drug half-life [62]. Various changes were made to adjust the surface area of the SLN using various techniques to achieve higher drug concentration and substantial permeability through the blood–brain barrier. Lopinavir SLN was modified using a hot self-nano-emulsion technique that involves a hot isotropic mixture of stearic acid, poloxamer and polyethene glycol in water with rapid cooling, which results in increased bioavailability relative to bulk lopinavir [63]. In a perfusion trial, a high level of positively charged or negatively charged SLN will result in a high cerebrospinal cortical volume that loses the stability of the brain membrane in rats. This helps to draw attention to the fact that a high amount of surface load change in the SLN will improve the adverse impact on health (**Figure 8**) [64].

NCL is a fashioned or customized SLN with a solid lipid matrix incorporated with liquid lipids with different fatty acid chains in a compromised ordered crystalline form that provides higher drug capacity. NCL consists of low-toxic lipid molecules that have hydrolytic and oxidative stability. It also indicates the biphasic drug release potential for a liquid lipophilic surface containing a drug and a solid center with a higher melting point for drug release through diffusion and matrix erosion [65, 66]. Preferential in vitro adsorption of proteins such as Apo E to the surface of DDI-loaded NLC stabilized using Solutol® HS 15 alone or a ternary surfactant method consisting of Solutol® HS 15, Tween® 8.0 and Lutrol® F68 in vitro suggests that these NLCs can be used to target Didanosine-loaded to the brain [67]. This approach can be a big advancement and is expected to greatly change the treatment of HIV. In fact, the ability to administer ARV medications to the CNS will make it easier to treat the AIDS dementia complex of HIV/AIDS patients and thereby improve their quality of life.

### 5.3 Inorganic nanoparticles

This class of Nanoparticles contains metal elements such as iron, gold, silver, titanium and silica that are currently used in anti-cancer treatment, molecular labeling of biomarkers, clinical methods, bioimaging, biosensors. Noble metal

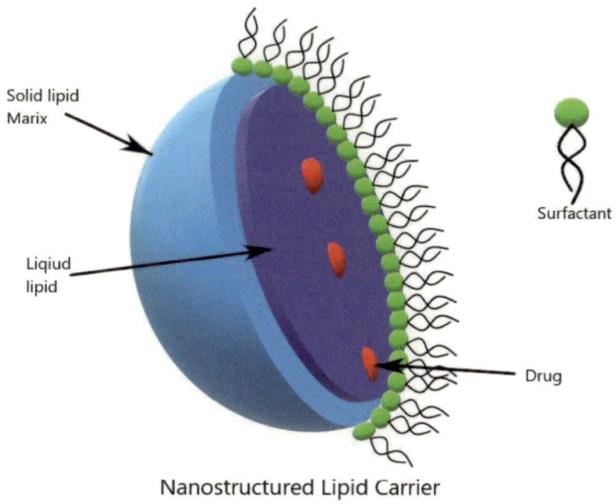


**Figure 8.**
*Pictorial art of nanostructured lipid carrier carrying drug.*

nanoparticles such as gold, silver, and platinum have been formulated using a range of techniques, such as chemical bio-reduction, rough mold, solution-phase synthesis, gas-phase deposition, and sol–gel. Silver nanoparticles are becoming more common due to their antimicrobial and antiviral effects against hepatitis B, herpes simplex virus, respiratory syncytial virus, monkeypox virus and HIV-1 in vitro, including clinical isolates and resistant strains [68–72]. Silver nanoparticles can bind to the gp120 protein and prevent viral entry, inhibit CD4-mediated viral fusion, and interfere with post-invasion phases of the HIV life cycle. Silver nanoparticles cause higher antiviral potency and therapeutic index relative to silver ion sulfadiazine salts [72]. Conjugated gold nanoparticle with TAK-779 and SDC-1721 which allow for better anti-HIV activity than its aqueous solution. Inorganic nanoparticles have limitations such as cytotoxicity, DNA damage, cellular apoptosis triggered by membrane leakage assay and LDH assay [73]. Inorganic nanoparticles usually harm the mammalian cells, because elimination of such particles from the living system is difficult and create cytotoxicity to the normal health cells with the infected cells. Some scientists are seeking to solve this issue with new ways to minimize cytotoxicity.

### 5.4 Polymeric micelles

Polymer micelles are nano-engineered block polymer materials that have core shells much like surfactant-based micelles and have been used to enhance permeability, aqueous solubility, chemical corrosion safety, controlled drug release, provide hydrophobic surface modification. Polymeric micelles are engineered as a hydrophobic heart and a hydrophilic shell that allows anti-HIV drugs to be trapped depending on their polarity. In addition, the surface properties of polymeric micelles, such as hydrophilic blocks, may be changed by docking antibodies or other chemical ligands unique to receptors found in diseases such as HIV-AIDS (**Figure 9**) [74].

A number of pharmaceutical scientists have formulated polymeric ARV-loaded mice, such as lamivudine conjugated with stearic acid-g-chitosan oligosaccharide mice, by esterification process that results in pH-dependent drug release, low cytotoxic activity, higher cell absorption of HepG2.2.15-infected hepatitis

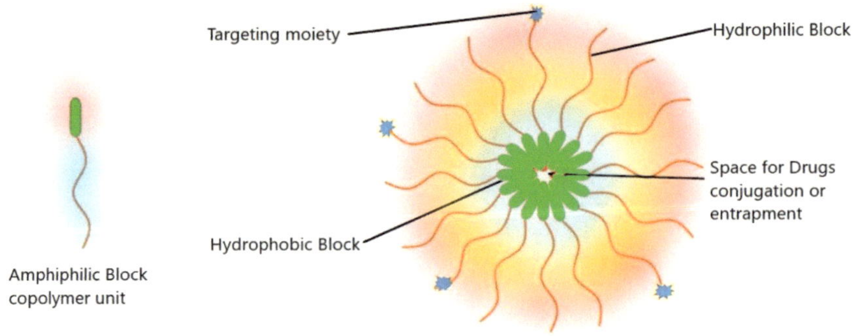


**Figure 9.**
*Pictorial art of Polymeric micelles.*

B virus-infected tumor cells [75]. Efavirenz polymeric micelles show substantial absorption rate and 3-fold improvement in the pharmacokinetic parameters of C-max from 1789 and 2657 ng/ml to 2856 and 7056 ng/ml in single doses between 20 and 80 mg/kg for healthy adult volunteers [76].

Copolymer: Poly (ethylene glycol) monomethyl ether and poly (ethylene phosphoric acid) (mPEG-*b*-PEPA) uses tenofovir, which varies in the length of the poly (ethylene phosphoric acid) chains and the degree of their saturation with tenofovir. Both adducts were found to be more active than conventional tenofovir against HIV-1IIIB in MT-4 cells; tenofovir 1:1 adduct with mPEG-b-PEPA49 displayed a 14-fold higher selectivity index. Thus, polyether–PEPA and polyester–PEPA block copolymers can well serve as scaffolds for the next generation of long-acting injectable antiretroviral formulations [77].

### 5.5 Nanocrystal

Nanocrystal drug itself may be a nano-sized drug particle that could be dispersed in aqueous or non-aqueous media. Drug Nanocrystals are mostly developed using approaches that promote a top-down approach or a bottom-up approach. Top-down techniques, such as media milling and high-pressure homogenization, are the most favored methods for the generation of nanocrystals because they are ideal for large-scale processing. Nanocrystal medication has longer colloidal stability, prolonged and continuous targeting due to expanded surface area. Nanoscale pure drug engineering is produced by means of an extremely hydrophobic drug that is strenuous to administer as an intravenous solution or by means of drugs with a rate of dissolution-limited oral bioavailability. Using a media milling procedure, Baret et al. formulated Rilpivirine nanocrystals of 200, 400 and 800 nm and inserted into mice and dogs via intramuscular and intra subcutaneous route and their pharmacokinetic activity was controlled. Experimentally, each therapy results in substantial detectable levels of rilpivirine up to 90 days in dogs and 3 weeks in mice suggesting success in long-term HIV prophylaxis. The author's analysis also indicates that the intra-subcutaneous route of administration shows a steady plasma concentration while the intramuscular route shows a criterion have been met as well as higher clearance. Rilpivirine amounts have also been observed in lymphoid tissues during treatment, promoting the absorption of nanocrystals by macrophages [78, 79]. Cabotegravir (CAB) is a newer drug class in the list of Viral Integrase Inhibitors, nearing to FDA approval, nano-formulated fatty acid ester CAB prodrugs administered to different strains of rats, monkey and various invitro model which,results better sustained plasma level for one year, increased drug accumulation at lymph nodes, blood plasma, liver, enhanced cellular uptake and nanocrystal prodrug stability in macrophages, slow drug dissolution rate which suggest better half-life [80].

## 6. Conclusion

An empirical application for anti-HIV therapy in drug delivery system lies in the potentiality of a nanotechnology. Development of ARV drugs through nanotechnology-based system such as Liposomes, dendrimers, Nanoparticles, Polymeric Micelles, Nanovesicles, Nanoemulsion offers efficient & wide targeted drug delivery with modulated pharmacokinetics, a higher therapeutic index as demonstrated by in vitro and animal's in vivo studies. These nano-systems provide prolong drug circulation, high bioavailability, drug stability, better permeability, bioaccumulation in known reservoir sites for HIV-AIDS. It also demonstrated the application of ARV nanocarriers to deliver drugs across the blood–brain barrier and other impermeable tissue to kill HIV virus. On the basis of HIV lifecycle, diverse nanocarriers are surface modified with different moiety to prevent viral fusion with intended ARV drug delivery. The majority of works done in the field of nanocarrier ARV drug delivery system incorporate a single ARV agent. So, this chapter tends to notice about the multidrug delivery system which involves a combination of drugs can lead to tremendous efficacious treatment and downgrading of resistance profiles. Hence, nanotechnology provides a multifunctional system for scaling up therapeutic approaches with innovative formulation to fulfill diverse biological requirements.

## Author details

Inampudi Sailaja[1], Manoj Kumar Baghel[1] and Ivvala Anand Shaker[2]*

1 Department of Biotechnology, Parul Institute of Applied Sciences, Parul University, Limda, Waghodia, Vadodara, Gujarat, India

2 Department of Biochemistry, Parul Institute of Medical Sciences and Research, Parul University, Limda, Waghodia, Vadodara, Gujarat, India

*Address all correspondence to: inampudisailaja@gmail.com

## References


[1] WHO (Global Health Observatory Data Repository 2019). Available at: https://www.who.int/data/gho/data/themes/hiv-aids Accessed on 16 January 2021.

[2] Wertheim, J. O., & Worobey, M. (2009). Dating the Age of the SIV Lineages That Gave Rise to HIV-1 and HIV-2. PLoS Computational Biology, 5(5), e1000377. doi: 10.1371/journal.pcbi.1000377

[3] Pauwels, R., & De Clercq, E. Development of vaginal microbicides for the prevention of heterosexual transmission of HIV. Journal of acquired immune deficiency syndromes and human retrovirology: official publication of the International Retrovirology Association, 1996; 11(3), 211-221.

[4] McGowan, I. Rectal microbicides: a new focus for HIV prevention. Sexually Transmitted Infections, 2008; 84(6), 413-417.

[5] Boggiano, C., & Littman, D. R. HIV's Vagina Travelogue. Immunity, 2007; 26(2), 145-147.

[6] Littman D. R. Chemokine receptors: keys to AIDS pathogenesis. Cell, 1998; 93(5), 677-680.

[7] McArthur, J. C., Brew, B. J., &Nath, A. Neurological complications of HIV infection. The Lancet. Neurology, 2005; 4(9), 543-555

[8] Arendt, C. W., & Littman, D. R. HIV: Master of the host cell. Genome Biology,2001; 2(11), REVIEWS1030.

[9] Chauveau L, Donahue DA, Monel B, Porrot F, Bruel T, Richard L, et al. HIV fusion in dendritic cells occurs mainly at the surface and is limited by low CD4 levels. J Virol. (2017) 91: e01248–e01217. doi: 10.1128/JVI.01248-17

[10] Wu L, KewalRamani VN. Dendritic-cell interactions with HIV: infection and viral dissemination. Nat Rev Immunol. (2006) 6:859-868. doi: 10.1038/nri1960

[11] Wallet C, De Rovere M, Van Assche J, Daouad F, De Wit S, Gautier V, et al. Microglial cells: the main HIV-1 reservoir in the brain. Front Cell Infect Microbiol. (2019) 9:362. doi: 10.3389/fcimb.2019.00362

[12] Stoddart, Cheryl & Reyes, Richard. Models of HIV1 disease: A review of current status. Drug Discovery Today: Disease Models. 2006; 3: 113-119.

[13] Lin J. H. Role of pharmacokinetics in the discovery and development of indinavir. Advanced drug delivery reviews, 1999; 39(3): 33-49.

[14] Musacchio, T., &Torchilin, V. P. Recent developments in lipid-based pharmaceutical nanocarriers. Frontiers in bioscience (Landmark edition), 2011;16: 1388-1412.

[15] 15.Mueller, B. U., Sleasman, J., Nelson, R. P., Jr, Smith, S., Deutsch, P. J., Ju, W., Steinberg, S. M., Balis, F. M., Jarosinski, P. F., Brouwers, P., Mistry, G., Winchell, G., Zwerski, S., Sei, S., Wood, L. V., Zeichner, S., &Pizzo, P. A . A phase I/II study of the protease inhibitor indinavir in children with HIV infection. Paediatrics, 1998; 102(1 Pt 1), 101-109.

[16] Rohan, L., &Mallipeddi. Progress in antiretroviral drug delivery using nanotechnology. International Journal of Nanomedicine, 2010; 533-547.

[17] Hammer, S. M., Eron, J. J., Jr, Reiss, P., Schooley, R. T., Thompson, M. A., Walmsley, S., Cahn, P., Fischl, M. A., Gatell, J. M., Hirsch, M. S., Jacobsen, D. M., Montaner, J. S., Richman, D. D., Yeni, P. G., Volberding, P. A., & International AIDS Society-US.

Antiretroviral treatment of adult HIV infection: 2008 recommendations of the International AIDS Society-USA panel. JAMA, 2008; 300(5), 555-570.

[18] Varatharajan, L., & Thomas, S. A. The transport of anti-HIV drugs across blood-CNS interfaces: summary of current knowledge and recommen dations for further research. Antiviral Research, 2009; 82(2), A99–A109.

[19] Redel, L., Le Douce, V., Cherrier, T., Marban, C., Janossy, A., Aunis, D., Van Lint, C., Rohr, O., & Schwartz, C. HIV-1 regulation of latency in the monocyte-macrophage lineage and CD4+ T lymphocytes. Journal of leukocyte biology, 2010; 87(4), 575-588.

[20] Li, S. D., & Huang, L. Pharmacokinetics and biodistribution of nanoparticles. Molecular Pharmaceutics, 2008; 5(4), 496-504.

[21] LaVan, D. A., Lynn, D. M., & Langer, R. Moving smaller in drug discovery and delivery. Nature reviews. Drug discovery. 2002; 1(1), 77-84.

[22] Amiji, M. M., Vyas, T. K., & Shah, L. K. Role of nanotechnology in HIV/AIDS treatment: the potential to overcome the viral reservoir challenge. Discovery medicine,2006; 6(34): 157-162.

[23] Kumar, L., Verma, S., Prasad, D. N., Bhardwaj, A., Vaidya, B., & Jain, A. K. Nanotechnology: a magic bullet for HIV AIDS treatment. Artificial cells, nanomedicine, and biotechnology,2015; 43(2): 71-86.

[24] Sharma, P., &Garg, S. Pure drug and polymer-based nanotechnologies for the improved solubility, stability, bioavailability and targeting of anti-HIV drugs. Advanced drug delivery reviews, 2010; 62(4): 491-502.

[25] Takeuchi, H., Yamamoto, H., & Kawashima, Y. Mucoadhesive nanoparticulate systems for peptide drug delivery. Advanced drug delivery reviews, 2001;47(1): 39-54.

[26] Langer R. Polymers for the sustained release of proteins and other macromolecules. Nature. 1976; 263:797-800.

[27] Sharma, A. Liposomes in drug delivery: Progress and limitations. International Journal of Pharmaceutics, 1997;154(2): 123-140.

[28] Jin, S. X., Bi, D. Z., Wang, J., Wang, Y. Z., Hu, H. G., & Deng, Y. H. Pharmacokinetics and tissue distribution of zidovudine in rats following intravenous administration of zidovudine myristate loaded liposomes. Die Pharmazie,2005; 60(11): 840-843.

[29] Chopra, S., Venkatesan, N., &Betageri, G. V. (2013). Liposomes as nanocarriers for anti-HIV therapy. Drug Delivery and Translational Research, 3(5), 471-478.

[30] Lasic DD. Liposomes in gene delivery. New York: CRC Press; 1997. p. 67-112.

[31] Makabi-Panzu, B., Gourde, P., Désormeaux, A., & Bergeron, M. G. Intracellular and serum stability of liposomal 2′,3′-dideoxycytidine. Effect of lipid composition. Cellular and molecular biology (Noisy-le-Grand, France), 1998; 44(2): 277-284.

[32] Oussoren, C., Magnani, M., Fraternale, A., Casabianca, A., Chiarantini, L., Ingebrigsten, R., Underberg, W. J., & Storm, G. (1999). Liposomes as carriers of the antiretroviral agent dideoxycytidine-5′-triphosphate. International journal of pharmaceutics, 1999; 180(2): 261-270.

[33] Jain, S., Tiwary, A. K., & Jain, N. K. Sustained and targeted delivery of an anti-HIV agent using elastic liposomal formulation: mechanism of action.

Current drug delivery, 2006; 3(2): 157-166.

[34] Kaur, C. D., Nahar, M., & Jain, N. K. Lymphatic targeting of zidovudine using surface-engineered liposomes. Journal of drug targeting,2008; 16(10), 798-805.

[35] Clayton, R., Ohagen, A., Nicol, F., Del Vecchio, A. M., Jonckers, T. H., Goethals, O., Van Loock, M., Michiels, L., Grigsby, J., Xu, Z., Zhang, Y. P., Gutshall, L. L., Cunningham, M., Jiang, H., Bola, S., Sarisky, R. T., &Hertogs, K. Sustained and specific in vitro inhibition of HIV-1 replication by a protease inhibitor encapsulated in gp120-targeted liposomes. Antiviral Research, 2009; 84(2), 142-149.

[36] Saiyed, Z. M., Gandhi, N. H., & Nair, M. P Magnetic nanoformulation of azidothymidine 5′-triphosphate for targeted delivery across the blood-brain barrier. International journal of nanomedicine,2010; 5, 157-166.

[37] Dubey, V., Nahar, M., Mishra, D., Mishra, P., & Jain, N. K. Surface structured liposomes for site-specific delivery of an antiviral agent-indinavir. Journal of Drug Targeting, 2010; 19(4): 258-269.

[38] Bronshtein, T., Toledano, N., Danino, D., Pollack, S., &Machluf, M. Cell-derived liposomes expressing CCR5 as a new targeted drug-delivery system for HIV infected cells. Journal of controlled release: official journal of the Controlled Release Society, 2011; 151(2): 139-148.

[39] Ramana, L. N., Sharma, S., Sethuraman, S., Ranga, U., & Krishnan, U. M. Investigation on the stability of saquinavir loaded liposomes: implication on stealth, release characteristics and cytotoxicity. International journal of pharmaceutics, 2012;431(1-2): 120-129.

[40] Asmal, M., Whitney, J. B., Luedemann, C., Carville, A., Steen, R., Letvin, N. L., &Geiben-Lynn, R. In vivo anti-HIV activity of the heparin-activated serine protease inhibitor antithrombin III encapsulated in lymph-targeting immune liposomes. PloS one,2012; 7(11): e48234.

[41] Dubrovskaya, V., Tran, K., Ozorowski, G., Guenaga, J., Wilson, R., Bale, S., ... & Wyatt, R. T. (2019). Vaccination with glycan-modified HIV NFL envelope trimer-liposomes elicits broadly neutralizing antibodies to multiple sites of vulnerability. Immunity, 51(5), 915-929.

[42] Tomalia, D. A., & Fréchet, J. M. J. (2001). Introduction to the dendritic state. Dendrimers and other dendritic polymers, 3-40.

[43] Svenson, S., &Tomalia, D. A. (2012). Dendrimers in biomedical applications—reflections on the field. Advanced drug delivery reviews, 64, 102-115.

[44] D'Emanuele, A., & Attwood, D. (2005). Dendrimer–drug interactions. Advanced drug delivery reviews, 57(15), 2147-2162.

[45] Witvrouw, M., Fikkert, V., Pluymers, W., Matthews, B., Mardel, K., Schols, D., ... &Pannecouque, C. (2000). Polyanionic (ie, polysulfonate) dendrimers can inhibit the replication of human immunodeficiency virus by interfering with both virus adsorption and later steps (reverse transcriptase/integrase) in the virus replicative cycle. Molecular Pharmacology, 58(5), 1100-1108.

[46] Bosman, A. W., Janssen, H. M., & Meijer, E. W. About Dendrimers: Structure, Physical Properties, and Applications. Chemical Reviews,1999; 99(7): 1665-1688.

[47] Jiménez, J. L., Gómez, R., Briz, V., Madrid, R., Bryszewsk, M., de la Mata, F. J., & Muñoz-Fernández, M. Á. Carbosilanedendrimers as carriers of siRNA. Journal of Drug Delivery Science and Technology,2012; 22(1): 75-82.

[48] de Las Cuevas, N., Garcia-Gallego, S., Rasines, B., de la Mata, F. J., Guijarro, L. G., Muñoz-Fernández, M. Á., & Gómez, R. In vitro studies of water-stable cationic carbosilanedendrimers as delivery vehicles for gene therapy against HIV and hepatocarcinoma. Current medicinal chemistry, 2012; 19(29): 5052-5061.

[49] Jiang, Y. H., Emau, P., Cairns, J. S., Flanary, L., Morton, W. R., McCarthy, T. D., & Tsai CC. SPL7013 gel as a topical microbicide for the prevention of vaginal transmission of SHIV89.6P in macaques. AIDS research and human retroviruses, 2005; 21(3): 207-213.

[50] Dezzutti, C. S., James, V. N., Ramos, A., Sullivan, S. T., Siddig, A., Bush, T. J., ... & Hart, C. E. (2004). In vitro comparison of topical microbicides for prevention of human immunodeficiency virus type 1 transmission. Antimicrobial agents and chemotherapy, 48(10), 3834-3844.

[51] Rupp, R., Rosenthal, S. L., & Stanberry, L. R. (2007). VivaGel (SPL7013 Gel): a candidate dendrimer--microbicide for the prevention of HIV and HSV infection. International journal of nanomedicine, 2(4), 561-566.

[52] International Organization for Standardization (ISO). Nanotechnologies —Vocabulary — Part 2: Nano-objects. ISO/TS 80004-2:2015 (2015).

[53] Panyam, J., &Labhasetwar, V. Biodegradable nanoparticles for drug and gene delivery to cells and tissue. Advanced drug delivery reviews, 2003; 55(3): 329-347.

[54] Blanco, E., Shen, H., & Ferrari, M. (2015). Principles of nanoparticle design for overcoming biological barriers to drug delivery. Nature biotechnology, 33(9), 941.

[55] Joshy, K. S., Snigdha, S., Anne, G., Nandakumar, K., Laly. A., P., &Sabu, T. Poly (vinyl pyrrolidone)-lipid based hybrid nanoparticles for anti-viral drug delivery. Chemistry and Physics of Lipids, 2018; 210: 82-89.

[56] Shah, L. K., &Amiji, M. M. Intracellular delivery of saquinavir in biodegradable polymeric nanoparticles for HIV/AIDS. Pharmaceutical Research, 2006; 23(11): 2638-2645.

[57] KUO, Y., & KUO, C. Electromagnetic interference in the permeability of saquinavir across the blood-brain barrier using nanoparticulate carriers. International Journal of Pharmaceutics, 2008; 351(1-2): 271-281.

[58] Meng, J., Sturgis, T. F., &Youan, B. B. Engineering tenofovir loaded chitosan nanoparticles to maximize microbicide mucoadhesion. European journal of pharmaceutical sciences: official journal of the European Federation for Pharmaceutical Sciences, 2011; 44(1-2): 57-67.

[59] Martins, S., Sarmento, B., Ferreira, D. C., &Souto, E. B. Lipid-based colloidal carriers for peptide and protein delivery- -liposomes versus lipid nanoparticles. International journal of nanomedicine, 2007;2(4): 595-607.

[60] Rawat, M., Singh, D., Saraf, S., &Saraf, S. Lipid carriers: a versatile delivery vehicle for proteins and peptides. Yakugakuzasshi: Journal of the Pharmaceutical Society of Japan, 2008; 128(2): 269-280.

[61] Chattopadhyay, N., Zastre, J., Wong, H. L., Wu, X. Y., &Bendayan, R. Solid

lipid nanoparticles enhance the delivery of the HIV protease inhibitor, atazanavir, by a human brain endothelial cell line. Pharmaceutical Research, 2008; 25(10): 2262-2271.

[62] Heiati, H., Tawashi, R., & Phillips, N. C. (1998). Solid lipid nanoparticles as drug carriers. International Journal of Pharmaceutics, 1998; 174(1-2): 71-80.

[63] Negi, J. S., Chattopadhyay, P., Sharma, A. K., & Ram, V. Development of solid lipid nanoparticles (SLNs) of lopinavir using hot self-nano-emulsification (SNE) technique. European journal of pharmaceutical sciences: official journal of the European Federation for Pharmaceutical Sciences, 2013; 48(1-2): 231-239.

[64] Lockman, P. R., Koziara, J. M., Mumper, R. J., & Allen, D. D. Nanoparticle surface charges alter blood-brain barrier integrity and permeability. Journal of drug targeting, 2004;12(9): 635-641.

[65] Abbasalipourkabir, R., Salehzadeh, A., & Abdullah, R. Characterization and stability of nanostructured lipid carriers as drug delivery system. Pakistan journal of biological sciences: PJBS, 2012; 15(3): 141-146.

[66] Zhang, X., Liu, J., Qiao, H., Liu, H., Ni, J., Zhang, W., & Shi, Y. (2010). Formulation optimization of dihydroartemisinin nanostructured lipid carrier using response surface methodology. Powder Technology, 2010; 197(1-2): 120-128.

[67] Kasongo, K. W., Jansch, M., Müller, R. H., & Walker, R. B. Evaluation of the in vitro differential protein adsorption patterns of didanosine-loaded nanostructured lipid carriers (NLCs) for potential targeting to the brain. Journal of liposome research,2011; 21(3): 245-254.

[68] Lu, L., Sun, R. W., Chen, R., Hui, C. K., Ho, C. M., Luk, J. M., Lau, G. K., &Che, C. M. Silver nanoparticles inhibit hepatitis B virus replication. Antiviral therapy, 2008; 13(2): 253-262.

[69] Baram-Pinto, D., Shukla, S., Perkas, N., Gedanken, A., &Sarid, R. Inhibition of herpes simplex virus type 1 infection by silver nanoparticles capped with mercapto ethane sulfonate. Bioconjugate Chemistry, 2009; 20(8): 1497-1502.

[70] Sun, Lova& Singh, Ankur &Vig, Komal & Pillai, Shreekumar& Singh, Shree. (2008). Silver Nanoparticles Inhibit Replication of Respiratory Syncytial Virus. Journal of Biomedical Nanotechnology. 2008;4: 149-158.

[71] Rogers, J. V., Parkinson, C. V., Choi, Y. W., Speshock, J. L., &Hussain, S. M. (2008). A Preliminary Assessment of Silver Nanoparticle Inhibition of Monkeypox Virus Plaque Formation. Nanoscale Research Letters, 2008;3(4): 129-133.

[72] Lara, H. H., Ayala-Nuñez, N. V., Ixtepan-Turrent, L., & Rodriguez-Padilla, C. (2010). Mode of antiviral action of silver nanoparticles against HIV-1. Journal of nanobiotechnology, 2010; 8:1.

[73] Braydich-Stolle, L., Hussain, S., Schlager, J. J., & Hofmann, M. C. (2005). In vitro cytotoxicity of nanoparticles in mammalian germline stem cells. Toxicological sciences: an official journal of the Society of Toxicology, 2005;88(2): 412-419.

[74] Nagasaki, Y., Yasugi, K., Yamamoto, Y., Harada, A., &Kataoka, K. (2001). Sugar-installed block copolymer micelles: their preparation and specific interaction with lectin molecules. Biomacromolecules, 2001;2(4): 1067-1070.

[75] Li, Q., Du, Y. Z., Yuan, H., Zhang, X. G., Miao, J., Cui, F. D., & Hu, F. Q. (2010). Synthesis of lamivudine stearate and antiviral activity of stearic acid-g-chitosan oligosaccharide polymeric

micelles delivery system. European journal of pharmaceutical sciences: official journal of the European Federation for Pharmaceutical Sciences, 2010;41(3): 498-507.

[76] Chiappetta, D. A., Hocht, C., Taira, C., &Sosnik, A. (2011). Oral pharmacokinetics of the anti-HIV efavirenz encapsulated within polymeric micelles. Biomaterials, 2011;32(9): 2379-2387.

[77] Nifant'ev, I., Siniavin, A., Karamov, E., Kosarev, M., Kovalchuk, S., Turgiev, A., ... &Ivchenko, P. (2021). A New Approach to Developing Long-Acting Injectable Formulations of Anti-HIV Drugs: Poly (Ethylene Phosphoric Acid) Block Copolymers Increase the Efficiency of Tenofovir against HIV-1 in MT-4 Cells. International Journal of Molecular Sciences, 22(1), 340.

[78] Baert, L., van 'tKlooster, G., Dries, W., François, M., Wouters, A., Basstanie, E., Iterbeke, K., Stappers, F., Stevens, P., Schueller, L., Van Remoortere, P., Kraus, G., Wigerinck, P., & Rosier, J. Development of a long-acting injectable formulation with nanoparticles of rilpivirine (TMC278) for HIV treatment. European journal of pharmaceutics and biopharmaceutics: official journal of Arbeitsgemeinschaft fur PharmazeutischeVerfahrenstechnik e.V, 2009; 72(3): 502-508.

[79] van 'tKlooster, G., Hoeben, E., Borghys, H., Looszova, A., Bouche, M. P., van Velsen, F., &Baert, L. (2010). Pharmacokinetics and disposition of rilpivirine (TMC278) nanosuspension as a long-acting injectable antiretroviral formulation. Antimicrobial agents and chemotherapy, 2010; 54(5): 2042-2050.

[80] Gauram, N., McMillan, J. M., Kumar, D., Bade, A. N., Pan, Q., Kulkarni, T. A., ... &Alnouti, Y. (2021). Lipophilic Nanocrystal Prodrug-Release Defines the Extended Pharmacokinetic Profiles of a Year-Long Cabotegravir. bioRxiv.

Chapter 6

# Employment as a Social Determinant of HIV Care and Prevention Outcomes

*Liza Conyers, Jen Yung-Chen Chiu, Sergio Rueda, Mark Misrok, Vickie Lynn and Erin McKinney-Prupis*

## Abstract

Advancements in HIV medicine have led to an increased desire and/or need to work for many people living with HIV. Despite the importance of work, relatively little attention has been devoted to specifically examining employment status as a social determinant of health. Unemployment/underemployment are associated with societal circumstances known to increase both the risk for acquiring and prevalence of HIV and other co-morbidity. Research indicates that being employed and use of vocational services is associated with positive physical and mental health outcomes. However, these positive outcomes can dissipate under poor or unstable work conditions. Transitions into or out of the workforce can also increase the risk of poor health associated with stress and potential disruptions or loss of access to critical health care. Given that individuals disproportionately impacted by HIV are also impacted by labor market discrimination, social exclusion, and poverty, there is an emerging sense of urgency to better respond to the employment needs of people living with HIV. This book chapter (a) reviews research related to employment as a social determinant of health, (b) provides an overview of the client-focused considering work model, (c) highlights key employment services, and (d) discusses implications for policy, service delivery and research.

**Keywords:** HIV, Social Determinants of Health, Employment, Unemployment, Quality of Life, HIV Care, Integrated Services

## 1. Introduction

People living with HIV (PLHIV) face numerous social and economic barriers including poverty, unemployment/underemployment, job insecurity, and lack of access to vocational services and education. Such barriers decrease their access to and retention in healthcare systems resulting in vulnerability to sub-optimal treatment adherence, poor clinical health outcomes, and poor quality of life [1, 2]. Because of the significant likelihood of job loss and/or underemployment after diagnosis, HIV can have a devastating impact on one's socioeconomic well-being [3, 4]. Although advancements in HIV medicine provide a pathway to end the HIV epidemic, many PLHIV are not able to access and/or stay connected to the biomedical and behavioral interventions needed to achieve viral suppression due to social determinants of health (SDH) [5] - social, economic, and political systems that can impact health risk and outcomes. The key indicator of HIV treatment efficacy, viral suppression, is essential to both improve individual health outcomes and prevent forward transmission of HIV. In recognition of the need to expand biomedical interventions to end the HIV epidemic, the United States Centers for Disease Control and Prevention [6] has adopted a SDH framework in developing interventions to address health-related disparities. SDH can be as broad as social, political, and economic systems, which are often referred to as upstream determinants of health, or can be more proximal indicators such as neighborhood, economic status, access to health care, housing, and employment among others. Although there has been an abundance of literature on a range of different determinants of HIV health (e.g., race, poverty, homelessness), there has been limited research related to understanding the role of employment as a social determinant of HIV health outcomes.

Since HIV is now considered to be a chronic illness with limited impact on life expectancy among those who have access to and engage in HIV treatment, many PLHIV are interested in starting or returning to work, to support themselves financially and contribute to society. Currently, living with HIV is as much about social integration and maintenance of independence as it is about optimizing access to medications and health care. Unemployment and underemployment are associated with societal circumstances (e.g., homelessness, food insecurity, incarceration) and activities (e.g., sex work, illicit drug use) known to increase both the risk for acquiring and prevalence of HIV and other co-morbidities; this complex, multi-layered context also creates significant barriers to health care access and employment services for individuals living with or more vulnerable to HIV. Within the context of these challenges, this chapter provides an overview of international research findings that highlight the relationship between work and health for PLHIV. We also describe the client-focused considering work model that was designed to help guide the complex process of exploring work options for PLHIV and highlight key employment service interventions. We conclude with implications for research, policy, and service delivery.

## 2. Employment as a social determinant of health

Rates of employment for PLHIV can be difficult to assess. According to studies in the US, Canada, and France, 45–62% of people with HIV are unemployed or receiving some form of disability assistance [7]. A nationwide population-based study in Sweden found that PLHIV were less likely to be employed than those who are HIV negative although the differences have decreased over time [8]. However, this study also revealed differential outcomes based upon key demographic factors (e.g., migrant status) and mode of HIV transmission (e.g., intravenous drug use). Another study examining the impact of foreign funding for HIV on employment rates found a 13 percent differential increase in employment rates for males in ten African countries that received the President's Emergency Plan for AIDS Relief [PEPFAR) funding compared to countries that did not receive PEPFAR funding [9]. This outcome was in contrast to a sharp decline in employment among females in PEPFAR-funded countries during the same time period. Overall, research indicates that the employment rates among PLHIV are lower than those reported in the general population [8]. These studies underscore that the heterogeneity of PLHIV as well as the political, social, and economic differences across countries can lead to wide variations in employment outcomes for this population. As such we need to better understand the relationship between employment and health, for the individual themselves, and for societies as a whole. The best way to minimize social exclusion for PLHIV is to promote (re) integration into the labor market for those who can, and wish, to work.

A systematic literature review investigating the impact of returning to work on health outcomes among the general population found that going back to work can improve one's health [10]. Longitudinal studies support the health benefits of return-to-work in a variety of populations and settings by showing significant improvements in health after going back to work or significant declines in health associated with continued unemployment. Cross-sectional and longitudinal research studies that examined employment and HIV health outcomes among different populations (including men living with HIV who have sex with men) attending tertiary care clinics in the U.S. and Canada [11] found that employment status was associated with both physical and mental health after controlling for clinical covariates (demographics, HIV-disease markers and psychosocial factors) and that these differences were clinically meaningful. Carlander [8] found that both satisfaction with psychological well-being and satisfaction with physical health were associated with being employed in Sweden. Broader HIV health outcome indicators include health-related quality of life (HRQOL), which is a multidimensional concept that includes symptom management, perceived physical and mental health role functioning, activities and participation, and life satisfaction. Research studies indicated that PLHIV who were employed had higher HRQOL compared to their unemployed counterparts [10, 12, 13]. Employment is a critical determinant of HRQOL as it is a source of financial and life stability. Other benefits associated with employment include better social functioning, handling of life difficulties, and health management [10, 13, 14]. One study that examined the impact of employment on mortality rates among people living with HIV who inject drugs found that independent of markers of disease progression, employment was associated with lower rates of mortality [15]. More recently, Ware et al. [11] investigated depression risk in men living with HIV and found that employment was protective of developing depressive symptoms over time but retirement, often a planned separation from employment, was not associated with an increased risk of developing depressive symptoms. These findings are consistent with conclusions from systematic literature reviews investigating the relationship between employment status and health in samples of PLHIV, which have found that employment is associated with better physical and mental health status [10, 14].

When considering employment status as a SDH, it is also important to consider the impact of unemployment and/or unstable work as both are associated with increased risk for PLHIV developing psychological problems such as anxiety, depression, suicidal ideation, and other psychiatric symptoms [16]. Decades of research has demonstrated a strong link between poverty and poor health outcomes among vulnerable populations [17, 18]. An HIV diagnosis can have detrimental effects on the wellbeing of PLHIV and lead to job loss or decreases in productivity. [2, 16]. Research that investigates the impact of employment transitions indicates that those who are on an upward employment trajectory (i.e., transitioning from unemployment to being employed) tend to have no changes or positive changes in health behaviors while being on a downward employment trajectory (i.e., transitioning from employment to unemployment) is associated with greater health risk behaviors [2]. When examining the impact of employment, one must consider how outcomes may differ by quality of employment. In a cross-sectional study in Canada, Rueda et al. [7] found that job security offers additional mental health benefits over and above participation in employment alone for men with HIV but not for women. Gender differences may be explained in part by differences in the structure of occupations and characteristics of jobs available to men and women. However, individuals who have jobs characterized by high psychological demands, low decision authority, and limited job security report similar outcomes related to symptoms of depression and quality of life as unemployed individuals [7, 19].

PLHIV who have temporary or unstable employment are at increased risk of death compared to those with stable employment [20]. Returning to work can also act as a barrier to retention in medical care and can lead to increase in stress and anxiety for some PLHIV [20–22].

Of note, negative employment outcomes (e.g., job loss, underemployment) are more prevalent among key populations disproportionately impacted by HIV, including racial/ethnic minorities, transgender, gay or bisexual individuals, people with substance use disorders, older adults, and individuals who were formerly incarcerated; these populations are also disproportionately impacted by labor market discrimination, exclusion, and poverty [2]. A qualitative study examining employment as a SDH among gay men and transgender women in the Dominican Republic, indicated that unemployment had a negative impact on mental health and overall well-being [23]. Survey research findings indicate high levels of HIV employment discrimination (e.g., exclusion in the workplace, forced disclosure of HIV status, terminations or unwillingness to hire or promote PLHIV) [2]. In a study examining the effects of quality of work on 339 PLHIV in China found that negative self-image and workplace discrimination were detrimental to employment quality; however, male and highly educated respondents were better able to use social and policy supports to increase employment quality compared to their peers [24].

In addition to the research on HIV health and employment, limited research exists that examines the impact of employment on HIV health and prevention outcomes across the HIV Care Continuum and the HIV Status-Neutral Prevention and Treatment Cycle. The HIV Care Continuum is a public health framework developed by the Centers for Disease Control [25] for monitoring the progress of PLHIV from initial diagnosis towards viral suppression. The outcome indicators are diagnosis of HIV, linkage to HIV medical care, retention in HIV medical care, medication adherence, and viral suppression [25]. The HIV Status-Neutral Prevention and Treatment Cycle expands upon the HIV Care Continuum Model to apply a continuum frame work to both PLHIV and those most vulnerable to acquiring HIV with the ultimate goal of eradicating HIV through combination antiretroviral treatment for PLHIV and pre-exposure prophylaxis (PrEP) for those most vulnerable to HIV. Review of the research indicates a strong relationship between employment status and outcomes across the HIV Status-Neutral Prevention and Treatment Cycle. Unemployment and underemployment are associated with societal circumstances (e.g., homelessness, incarceration) and activities (e.g., sex work, illicit drug use) known to increase both the risk for acquiring and prevalence of HIV and other co-morbidity; this complex, multi-layered context also creates significant barriers to health care access and employment services for individuals living with and at risk for HIV. A longitudinal study in Vancouver, Canada that examined the relationship between employment cessation and behaviors associated with HIV transmission risk among people who inject drugs found that loss of employment was significantly associated with increased housing instability, illegal income generation, and high-risk drug-use practices [26]. Furthermore, participants with lower long-term labor market participation had higher HIV seroconversion rates. The authors conclude that exiting the labor force is associated with increased economic marginalization and drug use behaviors that increase exposure to HIV. Preliminary findings from the National Working Positive Coalition – Vocational Development and Employment Needs Survey 2019 (NWPC-VDENS) also suggest that, for many, transitions from unemployment to employment are associated with individual and public health benefits, including a reduction in HIV-related health risk behaviors [27]. Another study indicated that not being able to work impeded engagement in HIV care among a sample of gay men and transgender women in the Dominican Republic [23]. Nachega et al. [1] conducted a meta-analysis of 28 studies examining the relationship between employment and medication adherence and found that employed research participants had 27% higher odds of adhering to antiretroviral treatment than those who were unemployed. Although there was variation across low, middle, and high-income countries, the results demonstrate the positive role that being employed can have on HIV medication adherence. Another study examining predictors of medication adherence in Tanzania found that unemployment was associated with non-adherence [28]. However, one study in Toronto, Canada found that being employed was associated with discontinuous HIV care [28]. A qualitative study examining the perspectives of PLHIV in Bolivia helps to shed some light on discrepant findings related to employment status and medication adherence [29]. Overall, participants in this study reported complex economic activities and challenges with the dual management of HIV and their livelihood [30]. To a large degree, their skills and workplace flexibility and support played a major role in the extent to which employment fostered medication adherence or not. Common challenges that study participants reported included reluctance to disclose HIV status, challenges getting permission for time off for medical visits, and challenges related to the limited hours and geographic locations of medical clinics. In light of the potential benefits and risks of employment on their health, PLHIV and their service providers could benefit from having a comprehensive framework to help guide vocational decision-making that carefully evaluates the impact of employment transitions on medical, psychosocial, vocational, and financial/legal outcomes.

## 3. Client-focused considering work model

Receiving an HIV diagnosis is a traumatic event and, similar to the diagnosis of other chronic illnesses, an HIV diagnosis can fundamentally alter employment and career trajectories. Unfortunately, research studies indicate that many people living with HIV and other chronic illnesses are not informed of employment supports and models that can foster engagement in vocational development and employment opportunities. [31, 32]. PLHIV, like many others with chronic illness or health conditions, face many challenges when exploring work decisions whether it be the decision to transition in or out of paid employment, changing jobs, or seeking volunteer work. To assist with this decision-making process, Goldblum and Kohlenberg [33] developed the client-focused considering work model for people living with HIV, which was the first of its kind to help structure key factors for consideration by PLHIV when contemplating changes in employment status.

In 2018, this model was revised to apply to all people with emerging or episodic illness [34]. However, the fundamental aspects of the model are consistent with a primary focus on the self-determined (i.e., client-focused) decision-making that integrates the transtheoretical model of change [35] to help illuminate the different types of work-related decisions, services, and resources needed when individuals are at different phases of considering work options: contemplation, preparation, action, or resolution. According to this model, the considering work process begins when a person feels a pressure to change in one of four domains: medical, psychosocial, vocational, and financial/legal. Medical advancements have reduced health-related barriers to work for many and research indicates that one of the primary motivators to work is financial need [2] Psychosocial pressures to change include wanting to be a role model for others and vocational motivators can include being laid off or opportunities for career advancement. Each of the domains of influence in the client-focused considering work model (CFCWM) reflect different SDH that have been studied related to HIV health including demographic factors such as race, ethnicity, age, gender, gender identity, sexual orientation, and education level all have an impact on PLHIV's health status and treatment outcomes [34]. Psychosocial factors include stressful life events (i.e., homelessness, food insecurity, abuse, intimate partner violence), social support, HIV self-management skills, and use of non-clinical support services. Medical factors include access to and retention in HIV treatment, and comorbidity with other health conditions (e.g., substance use disorder, mental health, kidney, hepatic, and bone diseases). Financial factors such as work earnings and overall income are associated with health outcomes as they are indicators of whether people have enough funds to meet their basic needs. These SDH are all interrelated. For example, psychosocial issues encountered by gay men and transgender women (e.g., family and/or school rejection) can lead to limited employment opportunities. Likewise, poverty can also limit career development and vocational options. When designing individually responsive vocational interventions for PLHIV, one must plan for the different needs at each phase of considering work as well as the medical, psychosocial, financial/legal and vocational factors that can either limit or facilitate social and economic empowerment.

Interventions during the contemplation phase focus on responding to the question: *Is any change feasible*? This could entail medical assessments, job accommodation reviews, and/or assessing the impact of work on public benefits and access to health insurance. If the risks of pursuing work exceed the benefits of working, work may not be considered a feasible option. At the preparation phase, the focus shifts to: *What kind of change is best*? The response to this question includes setting vocational goals and evaluating progress towards those goals as one prepares for changes in work status. Preparation may entail additional schooling or vocational training needed to achieve a vocational goal. The main focus of the action phase is: *How to achieve the goal?* This could entail sending out job applications or resumes and interviewing for positions. Resolution occurs when the individual is satisfied with their vocational outcome or no longer feels pressure to change. The process of considering work is often non-linear. As a person begins their journey from contemplating a change in work status to preparation, and/or action, several factors may lead to reconsideration of goals and desired outcomes and moving back and forth among the stages of change until resolution is achieved. According to this model, the considering work process is complete when the pressure to change has been resolved either through successful attainment of paid employment or other outcomes such as engaging in volunteer work or deciding not to make any changes [34]. The core value in the CFCWM is underscoring the importance of having access to the resources and support to make informed, self-determined decisions. Without a framework, one may not be aware of the wide variety of employment services and policies that are designed to help facilitate work for people with a range of health challenges and disabilities.

The client-focused considering work model has been applied to the development and evaluation of a number of vocational interventions including *Making a Plan* (MAP), an eight-week group intervention to help PLHIV develop and implement vocational goals. Outcomes from a study examining this intervention [36] indicated increased preparedness and progression towards vocational goal attainment, reduced vocational concerns, less hesitancy about returning to work. It was also used as a framework to evaluate an integrated housing and employment intervention entitled *Foundations for Living* [37] and an HIV prevention intervention for African American women: *Common Threads* [38, 39]. This model was also used to develop *Getting to Work: An Online Training Curriculum for HIV/AIDS Service Providers and Housing Providers* [40].

Conyers and Boomer [41] empirically validated the CFCWM on a sample of 1,702 PLHIV who completed the National Working Positive Coalition's Employment Needs and Vocational Development Survey (NWPC VDENS). As anticipated, items loaded on each of the four domains: medical, psychosocial, vocational, and financial/legal. However, the vocational domain had two sub-factors: vocational concerns and vocational confidence. This finding is not surprising given that social cognitive career theory [42] distinguishes vocational barriers from vocational confidence and the CFCWM highlights ways in which each of the domains can limit or facilitate decisions to change employment status. Overall, the CFCWM can be used to help structure and evaluate vocational interventions and training to help expand understanding of the SDH involved in addressing the vocational needs of PLHIV.

## 4. Key employment interventions

In addition to employment, engagement in vocational services is associated with positive HIV health and prevention outcomes related to the HIV Care Continuum. Researchers have identified that use of vocational rehabilitation and employ-ment services is associated with use of medical and mental health services, use of supplemental employment services, higher health-related quality of life, and reduced health-risk behaviors associated with HIV transmission [43, 44]. A program evaluation of an integrated employment and HIV prevention intervention for African American women with HIV, *Common Threads*, indicated that 95% of participants were more willing to share personal stories with family, friends, and community members after completing this intervention to reduce HIV stigma and to proactively educate other women about HIV [38, 39]. Additionally, many also reported positive vocational outcomes including skill development and participation in marketplace activities selling their crafts at national conferences [38]. In light of the diversity of communities and individuals most impacted by HIV and their varied employment support needs, a variety of employment service delivery models have emerged to respond to these needs over the years. The following sections discuss several employment services that have been developed and implemented to facilitate vocational development and work entry/re-entry among PLHIV.

### 4.1 Integrated employment services

People with emergent disabilities, chronic or episodic illness often experience multiple life challenges. For example, individuals often experience unemployment and unstable housing at the same time, as employment status and financial status often go hand in hand. In a large-scale longitudinal study in Canada, one-fifth of the participants with HIV had transitioned in and out of employment due to contextual barriers, such as unstable housing [7]. The intersection of housing, poverty, unemployment, and poor health outcomes underscores the need for integrated structural interventions to address these complex issues. To respond the multiple, inter-related challenges that many PLHIV face, a panel of HIV service providers recommended integrating employment services within AIDS services organizations [45] as interdisciplinary services are needed for PLHIV to enter/re-enter the workforce. Scholars also recommend the provision of client-centered, holistic services provided by an interdisciplinary team as most effective, including health practitioners, case managers, social workers/mental health professionals, peer specialists, and vocational rehabilitation professionals [46].

The Housing Opportunities for Persons with AIDS administration [47] recommends ongoing and comprehensive HIV services One of the structural interventions provided to eligible PLHIV is integrated employment and supportive housing services, which results in improved HIV treatment outcomes, mental and physical health outcomes, quality of life, as well as reduced health-risk behaviors (i.e., drug use; [48, 49]). For example, the Foundation for Living Program was a demonstration project funded by the U.S. Housing and Urban Development's Housing Opportunities Program for People with HIV that was designed to provide integrated employment and housing services [47]. Eligibility for the FFL program included expressing an interest in employment, being physically and emotionally ready to participate in vocational activities, actively engaging in HIV medical treatment, and demonstrating a need for housing assistance. Participants developed an Individualized Service Plan (ISP) and worked with an employment specialist to achieve their employment goals. Participants in the program also received housing stipends and housing services. The program evaluation of the FFL program indicates that among the 58 participants who completed reassessments, 44.8% gained or maintained employment, approximately 30% reported a decrease in the amount of their housing subsidy, and over 80% achieved viral suppression [27]. The reduction in the use of housing subsidies by some allowed the reallocation of these resources to other PLHIV in need of stable housing. Providing integrated employment and housing services to PLHIV is an emerging trend and additional research is needed to further evaluated the effectiveness of this integrated service delivery model.

### 4.2 Micro-enterprise employment intervention

Micro-enterprise employment has been used in low-income areas to help economically vulnerable populations to engage in income generating work. HIV prevention microenterprise interventions have been applied for diverse populations. The EMERGE Project is an experimental microenterprise intervention for African American young adults who were unemployed or underemployed and unstably housed. The intervention group received text messages with employment resources, business education information, HIV prevention information, and a start-up grant for $11,000 U.S. dollars, which could only be used for microbusiness essentials. Results of the randomized clinical trial study show that participants in the intervention group achieved better employment and HIV prevention outcomes [50]. *Common Threads*, the integrated employment and HIV prevention program, also has a component of microenterprising, identified as the Micro-Enterprise (ME) Circle. The purpose is to reduce the impact of poverty on African American women living with HIV by increasing financial independence. Participants are encouraged to engage in marketplace activities, such as selling their crafts at national conferences. Many participants reported positive vocational outcomes including skill development and participation in the Micro-Enterprising Circle [38].

### 4.3 Peer employment model

The integration of peer educators/providers in HIV prevention and care services has demonstrated positive outcomes and has been adapted in many countries [51]. A peer employment model has also been developed in recent years to empower PLHIV to be involved in employment within the HIV services workforce. Peers are defined as people who have shared similar lived experiences (i.e. men who have sex with men, people who inject drugs, sex workers), and/or community members [52]. White et al. [53] defined peer health education (PHE) as "teaching or sharing of health information, attitudes, values, and behaviors by members of the group who are similar." Peer interventions and education have been utilized in the prevention and treatment of mental health disorders, addictions, and chronic health conditions. Peer educators have been incorporated into HIV care and prevention programs since the start of the epidemic [54]. HIV peer workers provide a variety of services including health education, psychosocial support, community outreach, linkage to and support in medical appointments, and treatment adherence. The rationale of peer interventions and education is that peers can provide appropriate norms and people are more likely to emulate a behavior if their model is a realistic figure for self-comparison. Peers can also reach out to and develop access to PLHIV communities in ways that other professionals cannot. Peer training and workforce development has become more formalized as state and national certifications have been created in the U.S. In 2012, Georgia was the first state to bill for health and wellness services delivered by peer workers with additional states following with development of peer certification processes in 2014. Peer certification is fairly new in the field of HIV services. New York State began an HIV, HEP C, and harm reduction peer certification in [55]. Peer-delivered services in health and wellness programs have been eligible for Medicaid reimbursement in the states with peer certifications. This has led to the professionalization and expansion of the HIV peer workforce. Peer training and certification programs contribute to development of a broader, more representative HIV workforce better equipped to provide culturally responsive services, and can help expand vocational development and employment opportunities for PLHIV.

## 5. Implications for policy, research, and service providers and employers

Advances in HIV medicine and increased access to treatment have expanded both the possibility and need for PLHIV to engage in the workforce in every part of the world. Despite these biomedical advancements, addressing the employment needs of PLHIV and examining the impact of employment as a SDH is relatively new and has significant implications for policy, research, and service delivery.

### 5.1 Policy implications

The International Labour Organization (ILO) issued Recommendation 200, calling for national policies and programs on HIV and employment that facilitate workforce development, sustainable enterprises, and increased work earning strategies [56]. In response to this call, exploring the degree to which existing health care, workforce, and other social policies, as well as statutes and regulations, impact employment inclusion is critical. Policy changes such as reduced eligibility for public benefits for PLHIV need to be assessed to ensure that decreased access to programs supporting income, housing, and health care does not lead to increased engagement in work that negatively impacts access to and engagement in HIV care, ability to maintain viral suppression and quality of life. Global and country-level research studies in Kenya and Zambia indicate that PLHIV experience a high level of workplace discrimination, such as exclusion in the hiring process or the workplace, forced disclosure of HIV status, and employment termination [57]. A study in Singapore also reveals that the success of obtaining and sustaining employment is contingent upon maintaining confidentiality of HIV status [58]. Ensuring that disclosure of HIV status and participation in HIV testing is voluntary will reduce workplace discrimination. Policy coordination across sectors including public disability benefits, health care and insurance, employers, workforce development and vocational rehabilitation are needed. Peters [59] recommends the strategic coordination of policies across government programs that work to remove redundancy in programs or services and to close existing service gaps. Working together, policymakers, service providers, and PLHIV can outline and enact optimal policy changes related to program eligibility, income supports, and vocational opportunities for

PLHIV. People living with HIV who can work and want to work should not live-in fear of losing access to life-saving health care, treatment, or supportive services.

### 5.2 Research implications

Unfortunately, many policy decisions related to restriction of public benefits and eligibility for employment services are implemented with limited research examining the role of employment as a SDH. For example, there are limited studies that provide a better understanding of the unique needs of populations most impacted by HIV and that examine the impacts of variations in the quality of work settings and job demands on HIV care and prevention outcomes. More research is needed to fully understand the role of employment services, employment status and work conditions on reducing health disparities and increasing health and economic equity. Much research investigating the impact of work and health disparities on PLHIV has been limited to considering dichotomous outcomes: employed versus unemployed. This limitation is largely due to the absence of data related to employment in the majority of available datasets. There is a need for researchers and stakeholders to identify existing and new datasets and statistical models to better understand a) the mechanisms and pathways by which vocational development and employment services, and employment status, function as determinants of health; and b) the impact of work transitions on retention in care, treatment adherence, health outcomes, and on quality of life and well-being [60]. Integrating measures that would allow application of the client-focused considering work model to examine job characteristics, stages of considering work, and associations between each domain of influence is needed to better assess outcomes related to employment status, job retention, career advancement needs, and health, quality of life, and well-being outcomes. This framework could also be further developed and applied to program evaluation of vocational interventions internationally. Empirical studies looking at the outcomes of vocational rehabilitation, workforce development, and other employment-related services, as well as the associations with health, prevention, and quality of life outcomes are needed. In response to this need, the ILO supports research on the relationship between employment and HIV care and prevention outcomes to better understand the role that employment plays in the lives of PLHIV [1].

### 5.3 Implications for service providers and employers

Rather than maintaining a narrow focus on biomedical interventions, service providers need to incorporate a culturally responsive, trauma-informed, holistic approach that includes both reducing barriers that limit vocational development and employment opportunities and tailoring services to the complex interpersonal and social needs of those most impacted by HIV. Given the variation in employment challenges and HIV health and economic outcomes across different populations most impacted by HIV, vocational development and employment information and services for people living with or at greater vulnerability to HIV need to be integrated throughout HIV care and prevention services beginning at intake [60]. Service providers with a focus on HIV care and prevention are especially likely to prioritize awareness and elimination of HIV stigma, and could provide resources needed to support individuals' ability to make fully informed vocational development and employment decisions with focus on legal rights and protections, health and economic well-being, quality of life, and access to opportunities. To facilitate peer workforce development, standards, policies, and procedures for peer provider training, hiring and employment, fair compensation, mentorships, and professional development need to be established [60]. Furthermore, as PLHIV experience transitions into, within, and out of employment, service providers need to anticipate, assess, and address the impact of these transitions on health (engagement in care and viral suppression) and well-being. Career decisions of people living with HIV are often impacted by the threat of losing needed public benefits if work earnings impact ongoing access to healthcare, housing, food, and other critical safety net provisions for people with disabilities or chronic health conditions. As health improves, benefits counseling and advisement is an essential service for PLHIV who would like to work without the risk of losing supports necessary to ensure greater health and economic equity [60].

Disability policies must balance the potentially conflicting needs to provide assistance for those who could not work, as well as incentives for those who can work in a way that meets their essential needs [61].

Research in Malawi indicates that addressing HIV-related stigma in the workplace is critical to improving labor force participation. Sprague et al. [57] proposed the employment continuum framework, which addresses HIV stigma and workplace discrimination at various workforce entry points. Other recommendations include promotion of equity and inclusion in hiring practices, including establishing organizational policies that ensure non-discrimination and safety.

## 6. Conclusion

Advances in HIV research have increased the availability and distribution of antiviral therapy and have drastically changed the course of the HIV epidemic. People diagnosed with HIV who begin care and treatment early can now expect to live a normal lifespan, despite higher rates of co-morbidities than their HIV-negative peers [62]. These advances provide an opportunity for policymakers, service providers, and researchers, together with PLHIV and other stakeholders, to rethink the health and social services provided to this population. The public health approach has changed from caring for the dying in the 1980s to integrating health and social services that holistically support the health and well-being of people living with HIV. Today, we need to expand services to go beyond the medical model to include vocational and educational supports and provide supportive services for people living with and at greater vulnerability to HIV transmission. Vocational opportunity and employment supports are prevention and treatment interventions and can be adopted and implemented in existing community-based organizations and clinics that serve the health and social service needs of PLHIV and those at greater vulnerability to HIV. We now need policymakers and other stakeholders to recognize the need to develop evidence-informed policies to address the growing vocational needs of this population.

## Acknowledgements

The authors would like to thank Nia Staples for her technical assistance with citations as well as members of the NWPC Research Working Group for their ongoing work and contributions to this important area of scholarship. We would also like to thank ViiV Healthcare for their support with funding for the publication of this manuscript.

## Conflict of interest

The authors declare no conflict of interest.

## Notes/thanks/other declarations

The authors are members of the National Working Positive Coalition Research Working Group.

## Author details

Liza Conyers[1*], Jen Yung-Chen Chiu[2], Sergio Rueda[3], Mark Misrok[4], Vickie Lynn[5] and Erin McKinney-Prupis[6]

1 Department of Educational Psychology, Counseling, Special Education, Penn State University, PA, United States

2 Department of Educational Foundations and Counseling, Hunter College, City University of New York, New York, NY, United States

3 Institute for Mental Health Policy Research and Campbell Family, Mental Health Research Institute, Centre for Addiction and Mental Health, Department of Psychiatry, University of Toronto, Toronto, Canada

4 National Working Positive Coalition, NY, United States

5 University of South Florida, School of Social Work, Tampa, FL, United States

6 The Alliance for Positive Change, Inc, New York, NY, United States

*Address all correspondence to: lmc11@psu.edu

## References

[1] Nachega JB, Uthman OA, Peltzer K, Richardson LA, Mills EJ, Amekudzi K, et al. Association between antiretroviral therapy adherence and employment status: systematic review and meta-analysis. Bull World Health Organ. 2015 Jan 1;93(1):29-41.

[2] Conyers LM, Richardson LA, Datti PA, Koch LC, Misrok M. A Critical Review of Health, Social, and Prevention Outcomes Associated With Employment for People Living With HIV. AIDS Educ Prev. 2017 Oct;29(5):475-490.

[3] Mgbako O, Miller EH, Santoro AF, Remien RH, Shalev N, Olender S, et al. COVID-19, Telemedicine, and Patient Empowerment in HIV Care and Research. AIDS Behav. 2020 Jul 1;24(7):1990-1993.

[4] Massari V, Lapostolle A, Cadot E, Parizot I, Dray-Spira R, Chauvin P. Gender, socio-economic status, migration origin and neighbourhood of residence are barriers to HIV testing in the Paris metropolitan area. AIDS Care. 2011 Dec;23(12):1609-1618.

[5] HIV National Strategic Plan for the United States: A Roadmap to End the Epidemic 2021-2025. In Washington, DC: NHS U.S. Department of Health and Human Services; 2021.

[6] Center for Disease Control. Programs Addressing Social Determinants of Health [Internet]. Centers for Disease Control and Prevention. 2020. [Cited May 2021] Available from: https://www.cdc.gov/socialdeterminants/cdcprograms/index.htm

[7] Rueda S, Raboud J, Rourke SB, Bekele T, Bayoumi A, Lavis J, et al. Influence of employment and job security on physical and mental health in adults living with HIV: cross-sectional analysis. Open Med. 2012 Oct 1;6(4):e118–e126.

[8] Carlander C, Wagner P, Yilmaz A, Sparén P, Svedhem V. Employment by HIV status, mode of HIV transmission and migrant status: a nation-wide population-based study. AIDS. 2020;35(1):115-123.

[9] Wagner Z, Barofsky J, Sood N. PEPFAR Funding Associated With An Increase In Employment Among Males in Ten Sub-Saharan African Countries. Health Aff (Millwood). 2015 Jun 1;34(6):946-953.

[10] Rueda S, Chambers L, Wilson M, Mustard C, Rourke SB, Bayoumi A, et al. Association of Returning to Work With Better Health in Working-Aged Adults: A Systematic Review. Am J Public Health. 2012 Mar;102(3):541-556.

[11] Psychometric Validation of the PROQOL-HIV Questionnaire, a New Health-Related Quality of Life Instrument–Specific to HIV Disease.pdf.

[12] Reis RK, Santos CB, Gir E. Quality of life among Brazilian women living with HIV/AIDS. AIDS Care. 2012;24(5):626-634.

[13] Rueda S, Raboud J, Mustard C, Bayoumi A, Lavis JohnN, Rourke SeanB. Employment status is associated with both physical and mental health quality of life in people living with HIV. AIDS Care. 2011 Apr;23(4):435-443.

[14] Hergenrather K, Zeglin R, McGuire-Kuletz M, Rhodes S. Employment as a Social Determinant of Health: A Review of Longitudinal Studies Exploring the Relationship Between Employment Status and Mental Health. Rehabilitation Research, Policy, and Education. 2015;29(3):261-290.

[15] Richardson LA, Milloy M-JS, Kerr TH, Parashar S, Montaner JSG, Wood E. EMPLOYMENT PREDICTS

DECREASED MORTALITY AMONG HIV-SEROPOSITIVE ILLICIT DRUG USERS IN A SETTING OF UNIVERSAL HIV CARE. J Epidemiol Community Health. 2014 Jan;68(1):93-96.

[16] Dray-Spira R, Gueguen A, Ravaud J-F, Lert F. Socioeconomic Differences in the Impact of HIV Infection on Workforce Participation in France in the Era of Highly Active Antiretroviral Therapy. Am J Public Health. 2007 Mar;97(3):552-558.

[17] Williams DR, Mohammed SA, Leavell J, Collins C. Race, socioeconomic status, and health: complexities, ongoing challenges, and research opportunities: Race, SES, and health. Ann N Y Acad Sci. 2010;1186(1):69-101

[18] Zeglin RJ, Stein JP. Social determinants of health predict state incidence of HIV and AIDS: a short report. AIDS Care. 2015;27(2):255-259

[19] To Work or Not to Work: Combination Therapies and HIV - Eleanor Maticka-Tyndale, Barry D. Adam, Jeffrey J. Cohen, 2002 [Internet]. [cited 2021 May 3]. Available from: https://journals-sagepub-com.ezaccess.libraries.psu.edu/doi/abs/10.1177/1049732302238748

[20] Ferrier SE, Lavis JN. With health comes work? People living with HIV/AIDS consider returning to work. AIDS Care. 2003 Jun;15(3):423-435.

[21] Li AT-W, Wales J, Wong JP-H, Owino M, Perreault Y, Miao A, et al. Changing access to mental health care and social support when people living with HIV/AIDS become service providers. AIDS Care. 2015 Feb 1;27(2):176-181.

[22] Serrano A. "How am I going to work?" Barriers to employment for immigrant Latinos and Latinas living with HIV in Toronto. Work. 2015 Jul;51(2):365-372.

[23] Barrington, C., Acevedo, R., Donastorg, Y., Perez, M. and Kerrigan, D., 2016. 'HIV and work don't go together': Employment as a social determinant of HIV outcomes among men who have sex with men and transgender women in the Dominican Republic. Global Public Health, 12(12), pp.1506-1521.

[24] Yu Y, Chen Z, Huang S, Chen Z, Zhang K. What determines employment quality among people living with HIV: An empirical study in China. PLOS ONE. 2020 Dec 1;15(12):e0243069.

[25] Center for Disease Control. Understanding the HIV Care Continuum. National Center for HIV/AIDS, Viral Hepatitis, STD, and TB Prevention, 2019. [Cited May, 2021]. sAvailable from https://www.cdc.gov/hiv/pdf/library/factsheets/cdc-hiv-care-continuum.pdf

[26] Richardson L, Link to external site this link will open in a new window, Mammel M, Milloy M-J, Hayashi K. Employment Cessation, Long Term Labour Market Engagement and HIV Infection Risk Among People Who Inject Drugs in an Urban Canadian Setting. AIDS Behav. 2019 Dec;23(12):3267-3276.

[27] Chiu, Y-C, Conyers, LM, Maulsby, C, Misrok, M. Employing People Living with HIV in the HIV Workforce: Research Findings and Recommendations. Seminar session presented virtually at the 2020 National Ryan White Conference on HIV Care & Treatment Conference. 2020 August, 14. Online.

[28] Semvua SK, Orrell C, Mmbaga BT, Semvua HH, Bartlett JA, Boulle AA. Predictors of non-adherence to antiretroviral therapy among HIV infected patients in northern Tanzania. PLOS ONE. 2017 Dec 18;12(12):e0189460.

[29] Rachlis B, Burchell AN, Gardner S, Light L, Raboud J, Antoniou T, et al. Social determinants of health and retention in HIV care in a clinical cohort in Ontario, Canada. AIDS Care. 2017 Jul;29(7):828-837.

[30] Palar K, Martin A, Camacho MLO, Derose KP. Livelihood Experiences and Adherence to HIV Antiretroviral Therapy among Participants in a Food Assistance Pilot in Bolivia: A Qualitative Study. PLOS ONE. 2013 Apr 16;8(4):e61935.

[31] Koch LC, Rumrill PD, Conyers L, Wohlford S. A narrative literature review regarding job retention strategies for people with chronic illnesses. Work. 2013;46(1):125-134.

[32] Strauser DR, Jones A, Chiu C-Y, Tansey T, Chan F. Career development of young adult cancer survivors: A conceptual framework. J Vocat Rehabil. 2015;42(2):167-176

[33] Goldblum P, Kohlenberg B. Vocational counseling for people with HIV: The client-focused considering work model. Journal of Vocational Rehabilitation. 2005 Apr;22(2):115-124.

[34] Conyers LM. A client-focused considering work model for people with emerging or episodic illnesses. J Vocat Rehabil. 2018 Jan 1;48(3):331-343.

[35] DiClemente CC, Prochaska JO. Toward a comprehensive, transtheoretical model of change: Stages of change and addictive behaviors. In: Treating addictive behaviors, 2nd ed. New York, NY, US: Plenum Press; 1998. p. 3-24. (Applied clinical psychology).

[36] Kohlenberg, B. and Watts, M., 2003. Considering work for people living with HIV/AIDS: Evaluation of a group employment counseling program. Journal of Rehabilitation, 69(1), pp.22-29.

[37] Chiu Y-C, Conyers LM, Eissenstat SJ, Misrok M. Foundations for Living: Evaluation of an Integrated Employment and Housing Program for People Living With HIV. Rehabilitation Counseling Bulletin. 2020 Oct 1;0034355220962175.

[38] Chang, H-Y, Conyers, L., & Johnson, V. Program evaluation of a trauma-informed HIV prevention and vocational development intervention for African American women. Paper presented at the National Ryan White Conference on HIV Care & Treatment. Washington, DC. 2020 August 14.

[39] Conyers L, Chiu Y-C, Shamburger-Rousseau A, Johnson V, Misrok M. Common Threads: An Integrated HIV Prevention and Vocational Development Intervention for African American Women Living with HIV/AIDS. Journal of Health Disparities Research and Practice [Internet]. 2015 Jan 23;7(7). Available from: https://digitalscholarship.unlv.edu/jhdrp/vol7/iss7/9

[40] US Department of Housing and Urban Development HUD, Getting to Work: An Online Training Curriculum for HIV/AIDS Service Providers and Housing Providers; 2017 [Cited May, 2021]. Available from: https://www.hudexchange.info/trainings/dol-hud-getting-to-work-curriculum-for-hiv-aids-providers/

[41] Conyers LM, Boomer KB. Validating the client-focused considering work model for people living with HIV and quantifying phases of change of commitment to work. Disabil Rehabil. 2017;39(11):1087-1096

[42] Lent RW, Brown SD, Hackett G. Contextual supports and barriers to career choice: A social cognitive analysis. J Couns Psychol. 2000;47(1):36-49.

[43] Chapin, M. and Holbert, D., 2010. Employment at Closure Is Associated

With Enhanced Quality of Life and Subjective Well-Being for Persons With Spinal Cord Injuries. Rehabilitation Counseling Bulletin, 54(1), pp.6-14.

[44] Conyers L, Boomer K. Examining the role of vocational rehabilitation on access to care and public health outcomes for people living with HIV/AIDS. Disability and Rehabilitation. 2014;36(14):1203-1210.

[45] Office of Disability Employment Policy (ODEP). HIV/AIDS Employment Roundtable. U.S. Department of Labor; 2021 [Cited May, 2021]. Available from https://www.dol.gov/odep/topics/hivaids/toolkit.htm

[46] Audain, G, Bookhardt-Murray, LJ, Fogg, CJ, Gregerson, P, Haley, CA, Luther, P, Treherne, L, Knopf-Amelung, S. Adapting your practice: Treatment and recommendations for unstably housed patients with HIV/AIDS. Nashville, TN: Health Care for the Homeless Clinicians' Network, National Health Care for the Homeless Council, Inc. 2013. Available from https://www.nhchc.org/wp-content/uploads/2011/09/AIDS.pdf

[47] Housing Opportunities for Persons with AIDS (HOPWA). *Enhancing System Integration to Improve Health and Housing Stability Outcomes for Low-Income Persons Living with HIV/AIDS.* Office of HIV/AIDS Housing, U.S. Department of Housing and Urban Development. 2016. [Cited May 2021]. Available from https://www.hudexchange.info/onecpd/assets/File/IHHP-Narrative-Final-Report.pdf

[48] Aidala AA, Wilson MG, Shubert V, Gogolishvili D, Globerman J, Rueda S, et al. Housing Status, Medical Care, and Health Outcomes Among People Living With HIV/AIDS: A Systematic Review. Am J Public Health. 2016 Jan;106(1):e1-23.

[49] Rourke SB, Bekele T, Tucker R, Greene S, Sobota M, Koornstra J, et al. Housing characteristics and their influence on health-related quality of life in persons living with HIV in Ontario, Canada: results from the positive spaces, healthy places study. AIDS Behav. 2012 Nov;16(8):2361-2373.

[50] Mayo-Wilson LJ, Glass NE, Ssewamala FM, Linnemayr S, Coleman J, Timbo F, et al. Microenterprise intervention to reduce sexual risk behaviors and increase employment and HIV preventive practices in economically-vulnerable African-American young adults (EMERGE): protocol for a feasibility randomized clinical trial. Trials. 2019 Jul 17;20(1):439.

[51] Simoni JM, Nelson KM, Franks JC, Yard SS, Lehavot K. Are Peer Interventions for HIV Efficacious? A Systematic Review. AIDS Behav. 2011 Nov;15(8):1589-1595.

[52] Medley A, Kennedy C, O'Reilly K, Sweat M. Effectiveness of peer education interventions for HIV prevention in developing countries: a systematic review and meta-analysis. AIDS Educ Prev. 2009;21(3):181-206.

[53] White SW, Roberson-Nay R. Anxiety, social deficits, and loneliness in youth with autism spectrum disorders. J Autism Dev Disord. 2009;39(7):1006-1013.

[54] Miyamoto Y, Sono T. Lessons from peer support among individuals with mental health difficulties: a review of the literature. Clin Pract Epidemiol Ment Health. 2012;8(1):22-29.

[55] New York State Department of Health. NYSDOH 2015 Blueprint on Ending the AIDS Epidemic. 2015; Available from: https://www.health.ny.gov/diseases/aids/ending_the_epidemic/docs/blueprint.pdf.

[56] Sarfati H. Book review: International institute for labour studies

— ILO the global jobs crisis and beyond — world of work report 2009, ILO and IILS: Geneva, 2009; 117 pp.: 9789200149088, 50 Swiss francs (34). Transfer (Bruss). 2010;16(3):449-52.

[57] Sprague L, Simon S, Sprague C. Employment discrimination and HIV stigma: survey results from civil society organisations and people living with HIV in Africa. Afr J AIDS Res AJAR. 2011 Apr 2;10:311-324.

[58] Ho LP, Goh ECL. How HIV patients construct liveable identities in a shame based culture: the case of Singapore. Int J Qual Stud Health Well-being. 2017;12(1):1333899

[59] Peters B. The challenge of policy coordination. Policy Design and Practice. 2018;1(1):1-11.

[60] National Working Positive Coalition. Strengthening Responses to the Employment Needs of People Living with or at greater vulnerability to HIV: Preliminary recommendation. HIV and Employment National Convening, 2021, April 20-21. Virtual Conference.

[61] Jong PR de. Sickness, disability and work: Breaking the barriers — A synthesis of findings across OECD countries – OECD. Int Rev Für Soz Sicherh. 2011;64(3):115-117.

[62] Helf M, EditorMarch 13 E, 2020. HIV Life Expectancy in U.S. Now Matches General Population—With Some Big Differences [Internet]. [cited 2021 May 10]. Available from: https://www.thebodypro.com/article/hiv-life-expectancy-in-u-s-matches-general-population-with-some-differences